# The Art of the Heal

# The Art of the Heal

*A Health Executive's Guide to Innovating Hospitals*

Rubin Pillay MD, PhD

**To order additional copies of this book, contact:**
Xlibris
844-714-8691
www.Xlibris.com
Orders@Xlibris.com
846394

# CONTENTS

# INTRODUCTION

*It Is Not the Strongest of the Species that Survives
But the Most Adaptable.*

—*Charles* Darwin

Yes! Change is the basic law of nature. According to Darwin's *Origin of Species*[1], it is not the most intellectual of the species that survives; it is not the strongest that survives, but the species that survives is the one that is able best to adapt and adjust to the changing environment in which it finds itself. Applying this theoretical concept to organizations suggests that organizations, in whole or just in part, will need to transform their strategies, structures, systems, or processes to cope with a changing environment such as the introduction of new technologies, a shifting economic landscape, or new legislation impacting their field.

Industries change for different reasons. Sometimes, the cause is a crisis. The subprime mortgage meltdown, for example, rocked the financial-services industry. Institutions that had existed in some form for a century or more, such as Lehman Brothers, disappeared

---

1    R. B. Freeman, "The works of Charles Darwin: an annotated bibliographical handlist," in John Van Wyhe's ed. *Darwin Online: On the Origin of Species* (2002).

rapidly. More commonly, competitive dynamics (anchored in a variety of drivers, including product quality, performance, and cost) produce big changes in the competitive landscape over time—think about how Japanese competitors gained a share in the US automobile industry over several decades. In some cases, a distinct catalyst triggers a discontinuous change. The iPod, for example, transformed the music industry, just as the iPhone and its applications changed the game in mobile handsets, demonstrating the power of creative destruction. Healthcare is facing such a discontinuous change[2].

The healthcare industry's disruption is taking place at a time when the overall pace of change in the economy continues to increase. Two measures highlight this long-term trend of increasing "industry leadership volatility": the churn rate in the S&P 500 has more than doubled during the past twenty-five years. And the odds that an industry leader will lose its position during the subsequent five years—the "topple rate"—tripled during the twenty-five years from 1977 through 2002[3] and the two decades from 1989 to 2009. When an industry faces disruption, companies often fail to appreciate quickly enough the nature, extent, and velocity of the changes taking place. A number of reasons explain this failure. Often, disruptions start at an industry's periphery, among companies that provide specialized value propositions to different customer segments. In these cases, market penetration begins slowly, with barely perceptible impact. However, change can occur much more quickly when significant regulatory shifts alter the "rules of the game." The net result of disruption is usually a massive reshaping of the affected industry and its key segments—

---

2   https://www.mckinsey.com/industries/healthcare-systems-and-services/ our-insights/how-us-healthcare-companies-can-thrive-amid-disruption.

3   https://hbr.org/2005/03/the-faster-they-fall.

where the profit pools lie, who gets them, and through which business models. Entire parts of the value chain may be unseated or change in importance.

Disruptive change is now the norm for most industries and healthcare is no different. The healthcare industry is undergoing sweeping change. To emerge as winners, incumbents should learn from other industries that have faced similar upheaval. There are already early signs that the "topple" has begun in healthcare. In an analysis of a three-year sample of the financial disclosures of 104 prominent health systems operating 47 percent of US hospitals, Navigant Consulting[4] Inc. found broad-based and significant deterioration of operating earnings. Two-thirds of the health systems in the sample saw operating income decline from FY 2015 to FY 2017. Moreover, 27% lost money on operations in at least one of the three years, and 11% had negative margins across all three years. The total erosion for systems with operating earnings declines was $6.8 billion, a 44% reduction. The main cause: hospitals' expenses grew by 3 percentage points faster than their revenues from 2015 to 2017. To reverse this operating performance decline, hospitals must achieve both strategic clarities regarding their growth and transformation investments, and improved operating discipline in a markedly tougher environment. Hospital systems that can supplement inpatient revenue with new, diversified revenue streams are more likely to remain successful and enhance consumer value. These investments are generally less expensive than building inpatient capacity and can help mitigate inpatient utilization declines.

Healthcare has always had the hallmarks of an industry vulnerable to disruption. For more than half a century, healthcare expenditures

---

4    https://www.navigant.com/news/corporate-news/2018/hsom-analysis-2018.

have risen considerably faster than GDP growth. Furthermore, healthcare has not achieved the types of productivity increases that most other industries have experienced. In fact, healthcare ranks near the bottom in terms of productivity improvements since 1990—only better than the construction industry! For decades, rising healthcare expenditures have triggered industry changes like managed care and cost-shifting to employees. Nevertheless, cost and productivity pressures have continued to mount and have created an enormous impetus for innovations that drive better outcomes at lower costs. Many such innovations are now possible. For example, technological developments (universal mobile "end points," sensors, AI, etc.) make it feasible to manage chronic diseases more efficiently. On their own, the cost and productivity pressures would probably have been sufficient to produce major structural shifts within the healthcare industry. However, the added pressure from the changing regulatory environment provides the catalyst for even more changes to occur, and to occur more quickly.

If the experience of other industries that have undergone disruption is a guide, the healthcare industry will see many new entrants. Few are likely to survive, but some of those that do may become new industry leaders if they can couple innovative business models with strong operational efficiency. Who these winners will be in healthcare remains to be seen, but potential candidates include technology companies like Apple, Google, and Amazon and retail giants like Walmart and CVS. Companies that leverage information and insights to help patients make more value-conscious care decisions and companies that make more closely coordinated care delivery possible will prevail.

Consumers may well benefit from the innovations that healthcare disruption is certain to unleash—consumers typically do when disruptive changes arise. Incumbents, on the other hand, often falter during disruptions, for many reasons. Many incumbents focus on the status quo, have incentives that encourage profit-and-loss leaders to concentrate on near-term performance across existing businesses, and are hobbled by significant organizational complexity that makes major adaptations difficult. For most companies, it is also quite hard to create an effective strategic response to disruption. A robust strategic response requires an incumbent to navigate a change in business models—to strike the right balance between the new and the old at the right time—something an attacker does not need to worry about. For an incumbent, the scope of change typically requires transformation, and historically only 30 percent of organizational transformations succeed. Classic cases of disruption (when a company faces a competitor with a superior business model that results in markedly lower costs) ultimately call for a significant boost in the incumbent's competitiveness, which can be difficult to impossible to achieve, depending on the circumstances.

Responding rapidly to industry disruptions is hard. At most companies, the economic constraints of operating a business at scale hamper the ability to make changes "in flight." Many organizations are also prisoners of their past—and the more successful that past, the harder it usually is to make changes. Furthermore, rapid responses may be especially challenging for healthcare companies. Many parts of the industry are heavily regulated. Interactions among stakeholders (payers, providers, patients, employers, and so on) are often complex. Proud professionals everywhere have deeply grooved operating models and successful track records.

However, the market does not care about the past or about any of these constraints. Hospitals that want to navigate disruption successfully must get in front of it quickly. Navigating disruption effectively requires a healthy organization, a solid governance model, and—especially—leadership. Leaders need to take on two jobs: they must run today's business while creating the business of tomorrow. To do this, they should have a clear vision, based on solid insights, of the future. This vision should include the key present and potential market segments. Which of these segments do the executives believe will grow rapidly or become more profitable? Which ones will shrink? Questions like these are crucial because healthy institutions need growth—growth drives value, creates opportunity, and enables distinctiveness. Without growth, large companies find it hard to create value after ten years and are six times more likely to exit their industries than other large companies. However, the vision of the future must also be grounded in an accurate understanding of which market factors the company can control and which ones are inevitable. The executives can then attempt to shape to their advantage the factors within their control and avoid wasting time and money on inevitabilities.

Leaders should also be willing to make significant changes in how and where resources are allocated. After all, a strategy is only a theory until resources are allocated to it. In making the allocation, the executives should take care to ensure that they are not under-resourcing the new strategy. There is also a second danger the executives should guard against: at many companies, budget processes favor existing businesses over new ventures. Research shows that about 90 percent of all capital-expenditure allocations can be explained by the previous year's capital-expenditure allocations[5] and although all of the companies had

---

5    https://www.mckinsey.com/business-functions/strategy-and-corporate-finance/ our-insights/how-to-put-your-money-where-your-strategy-is.

detailed planning and capital-expenditure-allocation processes, those processes were inadvertently reinforcing the status quo.

If a hospital is to survive industry disruption, senior executives must increase its speed and capacity for transformation and innovation. They should note though that despite the imperative and their desire to innovate their hospitals, and the magnitude of the opportunity for innovators to both do good and do well, all too many efforts fail, losing billions of dollars along the way. But the good news is that health systems are uniquely positioned to drive the change that patients need. We deliver most of the care, know the complexity of that care intimately, and have trusted brands. Given the complexity of the healthcare industry and the data and privacy issues involved, understanding the complexities and scale of health care is critical to driving sustainable innovation and health systems are domain experts, as such, the onus is on us to disrupt from within, but do so deliberately and in partnership with the tech companies (big and small) who can propel them forward—and other health systems.

Yes, big tech has made multiple unsuccessful forays into health care over the years, however, they'll always be back. The opportunity is just too big. There will also, no doubt, be several high-visibility failures in the venture-backed health tech sector as well that will lead the industry to question the viability of disruptive models, their investor's commitment to health care, and more. We'll hear again that health care is too hard.

These companies represent the finest examples of learning organizations that take lessons from past failures and adjust. Typically, after retrenchments like these, learnings are assessed, capital gets more focused on winners, and the remaining disruptors who've survived become more effective. Out of these hard times come disruptive business models. Think Amazon (retail) and Google (advertising) out of 2001 and Airbnb (hotels) and Uber (transportation) out of 2008.

Health systems, in my experience, represent the finest examples of mission-based companies that are delivering health care for the public good. It should be a health system's mission to keep the transformation focused on providing compassionate health care for everyone—regardless of coverage or their ability to pay. I think the pandemic has made this mission even more important.

The thesis of NQ 360© is that established hospitals and systems have every opportunity to not just survive but succeed in the future. But to achieve this, they need to create a future-proof approach to innovation that spans the gamut of having the right strategies in place to having the appropriate people, structures, systems, and processes in place to drive organizational innovation. It is based on what big established players are doing right in terms of innovation and the patterns that they exhibit that create value across industries. It is difficult to single out one organization that has figured it all out, but they are all characterized by having reinvented themselves over and over again.

## The NQ 360© Framework

Before we get into the framework, it is critical to explain what I mean by the term "innovation." In the context of healthcare, I define innovation as "the act of creating value in response to opportunities aimed at improving health and healthcare through the conceptualization and deployment of novel solutions and unique resource combinations." It could manifest itself as new market-oriented products and services, the creation of new internal processes or production methods, and of course, new business models. It is therefore relevant to the entire organization and is not just the purview of the R and D or new product development teams.

Our NQ 360 Framework is a practically meaningful, holistic, integrated approach to improving the Innovation Quotient (NQ) of hospitals and health systems. Its four interrelated component parts include:

*Charter* encompasses three domains: *Purpose* which is the reason for the organization's existence, *Strategy* which are the initiatives that the organization pursues to achieve its purpose, and *Innovation Strategy* which defines the innovation approach.

*Organization* comprises three dimensions: *Structures* are the division of work and resources we need to execute our strategies, *Systems* are the tools we need to align behavior across our structures, and *Processes* are the series of actions or steps that we need to take in order to achieve a particular end.

*Competency* refers to the knowledge, skills, attitudes, values, and behaviors that people need to successfully perform a particular activity or task. We differentiate competency at the leadership, individual and organizational levels (culture).

*Linkages* describe the relationship amongst various components (people, enterprises, and institutions) that are key to optimizing the innovative ecosystem.

## The Aravind Eye Care System

The Aravind Eye Care System, based in India, is the world's largest provider of high-quality eye care. It is also one of the world's most incredible and revolutionary organizations delivering surgical outcomes equal to or exceeding those in the developed world at less than one percent of the cost, treating more than half of its patients free of charge, and taking no grants or donations. Aravind's success is so perplexing, that it has been the subject of several popular business school case studies. In this book, we will use the NQ360 Framework to explore Aravind's history and the distinctive philosophies, practices, and commitments that are the keys to its success.

When a crippling disease shattered his lifelong ambition, Dr. G. Venkataswamy (better known as Dr. V), chose an impossible new dream: to cure the world of needless blindness. In 1976, then fifty-eight-year-old and a retired ophthalmologist, he started with eleven beds in the living room of his home and recruited his extended family to join in his mission. This tiny clinic defied conventional logic, and today, the Aravind Eye Care System is now the largest eye care system in the world with more than four million outpatient visits and more than six hundred thousand surgeries and laser procedures annually. What started off as an eleven-bed hospital has now become the conglomerate, Aravind Eye Care System. Today, Aravind operates a growing network of eye care facilities (Aravind's eye care facilities include fourteen eye hospitals, six outpatient eye examination centers, and seventy-five primary eye care facilities in South India), a postgraduate institute, a management training and consulting institute (LAICO has worked with over three hundred hospitals in India and other developing countries, and has trained over two thousand professionals from seventy countries), one of the largest ophthalmic manufacturing units in the world (Aurolab products are exported to 160 countries around the world and accounts for a total of 9 percent of the global share of intraocular lenses), a research institute and eye banks.

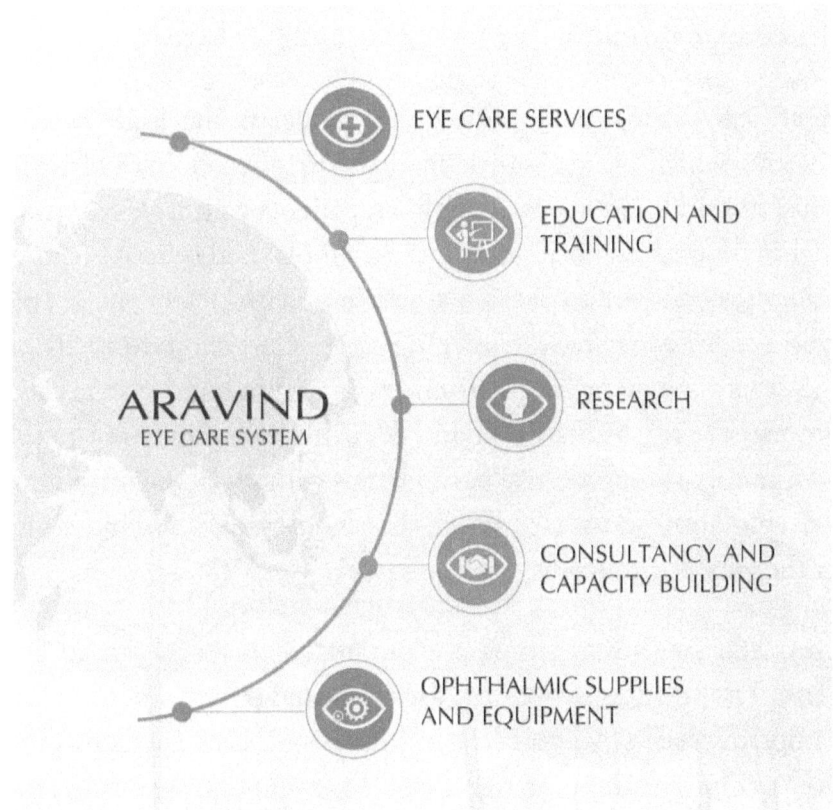

Source: https://aravind.org/our-story/

At Aravind, patients choose whether to pay or not. Millions are treated for free yet the organization remains stunningly self-reliant. Serving everyone from penniless farmers to the president, it delivers world-class outcomes at a hundredth of what similar services cost providers in advanced nations. Its model is emulated by organizations everywhere from Rwanda to San Francisco.

Aravind, with its mission to "eliminate needless blindness," has been able to achieve this by adhering to the principle of providing large volume, high quality, and affordable services in a financially sustainable manner both for the patients and for Aravind. Much importance is given to equity—ensuring that all patients are accorded the same high-quality care and service, regardless of their economic status.

A critical component of Aravind's model is the high patient volume, which brings with it the benefits of economies of scale. Most hospitals tend to focus only on patients who seek care from them or have systems to attract those who would otherwise go to other hospitals. In a situation where less than 15% of the people who needed eye care were seeking it, Aravind chose to focus on the other 85%—the "non-customers"—and to build systems and processes to reach them. Aravind does this by reaching out to the community through active partnerships with social organizations, local philanthropists, volunteers, the school system, and industries in the local community.

Outreach screening camps are organized to reach out to the general population, school children, and industry workers. These camps are visited by over half a million people each year, of whom over a third receive some significant intervention. Over time, the camps enhance the public's awareness of eye care and improve health-seeking behavior in the community, thereby growing the customer base for the hospital. About 2,500 outreach screening camps are conducted each year and these are highly standardized, resulting in increased efficiency and lowercase finding costs. The involvement of local community groups helps to build patient confidence and makes use of local resources, thereby reducing the cost even further.

More recently, a network of seventy-five vision centers was established with each center covering a population of sixty to seventy thousand. Patients "walk in" of their own accord and are referred to the "base hospitals" if they need cataract surgery. Through this combination of community-partnered outreach and vision centers, Aravind performs over a hundred thousand cataract operations each year. As a result of the awareness created through outreach and other means, another hundred fifty thousand cataract operations are done on patients who come to the base hospitals of their own accord.

A key factor influencing the uptake of services is affordability. This is best addressed by a holistic perspective that takes into account the total costs incurred by the patient, of which the hospital charges are a part. Besides ensuring that the hospital charges are affordable to the patient (which is a significant influence on demand), Aravind also addresses the other costs incurred by the patient in the way the services are designed and provided.

The following strategies to reduce travel and the associated costs and effort (what we call patient costs) have been employed:

- Eye care is made locally available through outreach and vision centers, which greatly reduces travel and associated costs.
- All investigations are made during a single visit, eliminating the need for the patient to make multiple visits and thus reducing travel and associated costs.
- Patients are offered a surgery slot immediately if surgery is indicated. There is no waiting list. This enables patients to complete the entire care cycle in a single visit.

- Prescribed medicines or spectacles are made available locally and at a fair price.
- Free transportation is offered to all patients identified during outreach as needing surgery. The patients are accompanied to the hospital and back by Aravind staff or a community volunteer.

# CHAPTER 1

## Charter
## From Vision to Purpose

*There is one quality which one must possess to win,*
*and that is definiteness of purpose, the knowledge of*
*what one wants, and a burning desire to possess it.*
*—Napoleon Hill*

Historically, an organization's charter was enshrined in its vision and mission statements. The vision statement describes what the organization will look like in the future while a mission statement describes how the organization will get there. Fundamentally, these served as a guiding beacon that depicts the kind of future to which the organization aspires and also provides direction to everyone in the organization as they focus their efforts on achieving the vision. Below are examples of vision statements of some of the leading hospitals and health systems in the United States of America.

*"Striving to be the world's leader in patient experience, clinical outcomes, research, and education."*

*"Will be a global medical and academic leader who will change and save lives."*

*"To become the Preferred Academic Medical Center of the 21st Century."*

The common thread that runs through all of them is that they are all similar formulations about being among the leading organizations in their industry. It's all about "winning," "beating the competition," and being "number one." Well, inherent in this approach to vision setting is that the organization is operating with a finite time horizon and mindset that there is an endpoint— becoming "number 1" or being the "best." This default win-lose mode can sometimes work for the short term but can have grave consequences in the longer term. James Carse[6] calls this leading with a finite mindset. A finite game is played for the purpose of winning—to beat a competitor. Finite games are those instrumental activities like sports and politics in which the participants obey rules, recognize boundaries, and announce winners and losers.

The consequences of this transactional approach are all too familiar: growing shareholder value as opposed to the needs of employees and customers, layoffs to meet arbitrary projections, cutthroat work environments, unethical business practices, and the rewarding of self-centered team members and self-serving leaders, amongst others. This leads to all kinds of problems, the most common of which include the decline of trust, cooperation, discretionary effort, morale, innovation, and ultimately performance. Finite players can never win an infinite game.

---

6    James P. Carse, *Finite and Infinite Games*, New York: Ballantine Books (1987).

Carse says that the infinite game exists solely for the purpose of continuing the game. There's no such thing as winning. There's only ahead and behind. The playing field is undefined and progress is hard to measure. Opponents change frequently as does the game itself. There are no clear winners or losers in the infinite game. Competitors drop out of the infinite game when they lose the will or resources to stop playing. The goal is to outlast your competition. Leaders who embrace an infinite mindset—where the game of business has no finish line—build organizations that are strong enough and healthy enough to stay in the game for generations to come and where the true value of the organization cannot be measured by the success it has achieved on a set of arbitrary metrics over arbitrary timeframes.

According to Simon Sinek, in the volatile, uncertain, complex, and ambiguous new health economy, the most successful leaders and organizations need to play the infinite game, not the finite one.[7] Playing the infinite game requires leaders to prioritize their purpose above anything else. Ultimately, we are competing against ourselves, and our success or failure should be measured against our purpose. Our competitors may push us to improve our products, services, marketing, etc., but in the infinite game, we are constantly striving to become a better version of ourselves in order to fulfill our purpose. Leaders should be willing to stand up to the pressures of shareholder demands for a focus on the bottom line, and stay true to their cause. They should be driven not to beat the quarter but to continue to improve access and quality and reduce costs. This is the fundamental difference between a finite "vision" based approach and an infinite "purpose-driven" approach. A vision describes what these hospitals and systems want to become rather than the change they want to achieve. It's

7    Simon Sinek, *The Infinite Game*, Portfolio/Penguin (2019).

time that we move on from vision and mission statements as the essential precursor to effective strategic management and consider organizational purpose instead.

## Purpose

Highly innovative organizations are not simply focused on delivering products and services for profit or shareholder value creation, but also have an underlying purpose to positively impact the world. Social movements, rapidly growing organizations, and remarkable breakthroughs in science and technology all have something in common—they're often byproducts of a deeply unifying purpose defined as "a concrete goal or objective for the firm that reaches beyond profit maximization."[8] It's a narrative that employees and customers can understand and identify with, to motivate them and counter the biases that would otherwise hold them back. A crucial aspect of purpose is its inherent intangibility. An organization's purpose is not a formal announcement, but instead a set of common beliefs that are held by and guide the actions of employees. We consider companies with a strong purpose to be those in which employees in aggregate have a strong sense of the meaningfulness and collective impact of their work.

Practitioners, including CEOs, consultants, and the press have long articulated their purpose within their organizations. Dennis Bakke, the CEO of AES, a global electric utility, alludes to the purpose of AES as "meeting the world's need for safe, clean, reliable, and economically-priced electricity." The Brazilian cosmetics firm

---

8    Claudine Madras Gartenberg and Andrea Prat and George Serafeim, "Corporate Purpose and Financial Performance," *Organization Science, Forthcoming* (October 9, 2018), https://ssrn.com/abstract=2840005 or http://dx.doi.org/10.2139/ssrn.2840005.

Natura[9] and the Danish pharmaceutical firm Novo Nordisk[10], two of the most successful companies in terms of stock price performance in the last decade, have explicitly stated a purpose beyond profit maximization since their founding. Richard Branson, CEO of Virgin Group has said, "It's always been my objective to create businesses with a defined purpose beyond just making money . . . our newest investment in OneWeb is also very much a purpose-driven business, looking to create a constellation of satellites to bring connectivity and communications to billions." [11] Similarly, Paul Polman, CEO of Unilever, has long supported the importance of purpose in business, "We have committed to help provide good hygiene, safe drinking water, and better sanitation for the millions of people around the world. It is about opportunity and aligning our purpose in business with this opportunity."[12] In these examples, the *purpose* is a meaning-rich articulation of the main business of the firm.

In academic literature, various definitions of purpose have been offered over time. One set of definitions explicitly focuses on a social objective for the firm. For example, Bartlett and Ghoshal [13] define purpose as "the statement of a company's moral response to its broadly defined responsibilities, not an amoral plan for

9    http://www.managementexchange.com/story/innovation-in-well-being.

10   http://www.managementexchange.com/story/how-novo-nordisk's-corporate-dna-drives-innovation.

11   "How to manifest purpose in business," https://www.virgin.com/richard-branson/how-to-manifest-purpose-in-business.

12   "Redefining Business Purpose: Driving Societal and Systems Transformation," http://www.huffingtonpost.com/paul-polman/redefining-business-purpo_b_6549956.html,

13   C. A. Bartlett and S. Ghoshal, "Changing the role of top management: Beyond strategy to purpose," *Harvard Business Review* 72, no. 6 (1994): 79–88.

exploiting a commercial opportunity." Thakor and Quinn[14] similarly define it as "something that is perceived as producing a social benefit over and above the tangible pecuniary payoff that is shared by the principal and the agent."

Purpose, however, need not be explicitly pro-social. Oxford Dictionaries define purpose as "the reason for which something is done or created or for which something exists."[15] Applying this general definition to a firm context, the purposeful company report—written by a consortium of academics studying purpose in businesses—defines the purpose of a company as "its reason for being."[16] Similarly, Henderson and Van den Steen[17] write that purpose is "a concrete goal or objective for the firm that reaches beyond profit maximization." We adopt this broader view of corporate purpose, as a set of beliefs about the meaning of a firm's work beyond quantitative measures of financial performance

Most established hospitals and health systems have no transformative purpose. They all want to be the "leaders" or the "best." Such a vision is not very ambitious nor motivational because it does not speak to us as human beings. It does not contain a strong narrative. The newer generation of employees is more interested in what a hospital stands for than its journey to becoming the biggest or the best. This is also increasingly reflected

---

14   , A. V. Thakor and R. E. Quinn, "The economics of higher purpose," ECGI-Finance Working Paper 395 (2013).

15   http://www.oxforddictionaries.com/us/definition/american_english/purpos.

16   The Purposeful Company Interim Report (May 2016), http://www.biginnovationcentre.com/media/uploads/pdf/The%20Purposeful%20Company%20Interim%20Report.pdf.

17   R. Henderson and E. Van den Steen, "Why Do Firms Have 'Purpose'? The Firm's Role as a Carrier of Identity and Reputation," *The American Economic Review* 105, no. 5 (2015): 326–330.

in the younger generation- millennials. A recent study[18] showed that 76% of millennials were willing to be paid lower salaries to work for a company that makes a difference in the world and nearly two-thirds (64%) won't take a job if a potential employer doesn't have strong corporate social responsibility! Millennials are quite clearly showing an orientation toward seeking meaning and purpose in their lives and are becoming aspirational, and as such will be drawn as customers, employers, and investors to equally aspirational organizations—this is to companies with a purpose!

Several other analyses support how important it is for an organization to have a higher purpose. The 2014 Deloitte Core Beliefs and Culture[19] Survey showed that businesses with a strong sense of purpose are more confident about their growth prospects, experience higher levels of confidence among stakeholders, and are more focused on long-term growth. Eighty-three percent of respondents who work for an organization with a strong sense of purpose are much more optimistic about their ability to stay ahead of industry disruption (versus 42% who do not have a strong sense of purpose) and to outperform their competition (79% versus 47%). These findings highlight the connection between a sense of purpose and the confidence required to sustain a successful enterprise.

Similarly, when George Serafeim[20] and his coauthors analyzed the 450,000 responses to the "Great Places to Work" survey, they found a direct correlation between the experience of a higher purpose

18  http://www.conecomm.com/news-blog/2016-cone-communications-millennial-employee-engagement-study-press-release.

19  https://www2.deloitte.com/content/dam/Deloitte/us/Documents/about-deloitte/us-leadership-2014-core-beliefs-culture-survey-040414.pdf.

20  https://ssrn.com/abstract=2840005.

and the economic results of that organization. Conversely, they did not see a correlation with a culture of camaraderie suggesting that higher purpose was a better predictor of firm performance than friendly work culture.

## Creating a Purpose-Driven Organization

Admittedly, the concept of higher purpose does not fit into most leaders' typical economic understanding of a firm. A higher purpose is not about economic exchanges. It reflects something more aspirational. It explains how the people involved with an organization are making a difference, gives them a sense of meaning, and draws their support. A leader's most important job is "to connect the people to their purpose."

When organizations fail to generate economic (shareholder) value, it is almost always attributed to a lack of commitment from employees. They were not very engaged and just went through the motions. They couldn't break free of old, tired behaviors. They weren't bringing their smarts and creativity to their jobs. They weren't performing up to their potential!

If like many executives, you're applying conventional economic logic, you view your employees as self-interested agents and design your organizational practices and culture accordingly. You provide training, incentives, and increased managerial oversight, very often with disappointing results. So you now face a choice: you can double down on that approach, on the assumption that you just need more or stricter controls to achieve the desired impact. Or you can align the organization with an authentic higher purpose that intersects with your business interests and helps guide your decisions. If you succeed in doing the latter, your people will try new things, move into deep learning, take risks, and make surprising contributions. Forging a stronger link between the business goals and the higher purpose of the organization increases the agent's intrinsic motivation to exert effort, diminishing the need for exclusive reliance on extrinsic rewards, and when an authentic purpose permeates business strategy and decision making, the personal good and the collective good become one. Positive peer pressure kicks in, and employees are reenergized. Collaboration increases, learning accelerates, and performance climbs. People who find meaning in their work don't hoard their energy and dedication. They give them freely, defying conventional economic assumptions about self-interest. They grow rather than stagnate. They do more—and they do it better.

You can build a purpose-driven healthcare organization by following eight essential steps:[21]

## 1. Envision an inspired workforce

It all starts by shedding the standard economic model for describing an organization's relationships with its workers which posits that the agent is effort averse. Since effort is personally costly, the agent underperforms in providing it unless the principal puts contractual incentives and control systems in place to counter that tendency. One way to change that perception is to expose leaders to positive exceptions to the rule. Purpose-driven employees, teams, and units exist. Look for them and examine the purpose that drives their excellence and imagine your entire workforce this way.

---

21  https://hbr.org/2018/07/creating-a-purpose-driven-organization.

## 2. Discover the purpose

Unlike a vision or mission statement, you cannot invent a higher purpose, it already exists. You can discover it through empathy—by feeling and understanding the deepest common needs of your workforce. That involves asking provocative questions, listening, and reflecting. Why does your organization exist? What motivates you to do the work that you do? What is the greatest possible impact you can make on the lives of others through your work? Why is this important? And ask these questions five times: it's a technique called the Five Whys. Imagine a person asking you, "Why does your organization exist?" What would you say? After thinking about your answer, they then asked you, "Why is that important?" What would you say next? And as they continued to probe further and further, asking again and again, "Why is that important?" What layers of purpose and meaning reveal themselves?

Now use the opposite approach, and ask your people, "What single word is the bull's-eye of the bull's-eye, the focus of the focus, the center of the center, the very essence of your organization?" Even though this is not your purpose statement, it is the single-word focus of your organization. And through the process of elimination, find that a single word may take several attempts with your people. One single word will bring meaning to every organization's meetings: employee, customer, and supplier relationships. It will be the essence, the single word that brings meaningful work to everything you do.

The next step is to ask, "Instead of having one word, what three words would you use to focus your people's energies on?" Now write a simple, non-technical three-word phrase that everyone can clearly understand that becomes your purpose statement. Refine your purpose statement so that when someone asks you what is your organization about, you can simply say, "The reason we exist is to . . ."

If you are still unsure of whether the purpose will provide direction for your work, inspire the team to sacrifice and endure beyond your lifetimes, it has to meet five standards:[22]

**For something**: affirmative and optimistic (e.g., not against illness and disease but *for* wellness)

**Inclusive**: open to all those who would like to contribute. Innately we want to belong (e.g., inspire communities by connecting people)

**Service-oriented**: for the primary benefit of others (not company-focused benefits))

**Resilient**: able to endure political, technological, and socio-cultural change (not product or service driven but cause-driven)

**Idealistic**: big, bold, and ultimately unachievable

Once you have discovered your organization's purpose, now ask each individual that is involved in the process to independently answer the following questions.

Yes/No: Do you find this purpose personally inspiring?

Yes/No: Can you envision this purpose being as valid 100 years from now as it is today?

---

22  Simon Sinek, *The Infinite Game* (2019), Portfolio/Penguin.

Yes/No: Does the purpose help you think expansively about the long-term possibilities and range of activities the organization can consider over the next 100 years, beyond its current products, services, markets, industries, and strategies?

Yes/No: Does the purpose help you to decide what activities to not pursue, to eliminate from consideration?

Yes/No: Is this purpose authentic—something true to what the organization is all about–not merely words on paper that "sound nice?"

Yes/No: Would this purpose be greeted with enthusiasm rather than cynicism by a broad base of people in the organization?

Yes/No: When telling your children and/or other loved ones what you do for a living, would you feel proud in describing your work in terms of this purpose?

If most of your people (at least 80 to 90 percent) answer yes to all of the questions above, then you can confidently move forward with your new purpose statement. If not, then you need to keep working through the process until you have widespread alignment around these questions. Defining the purpose of your organization is hard work, but the results are worth it!

### 3. Aspire for Authenticity

When an organization announces its purpose and values, but the words don't govern the behavior of senior leadership, they ring hollow. Everyone recognizes the hypocrisy, and employees become more cynical. The process does harm. The assumption that people act only out of self-interest also gets applied to leaders, who are often seen as disingenuous if they claim other motivations. So identify a purpose and a set of values, and live them with integrity. If your purpose is authentic, people know, because it drives every decision and you do things other companies would not.

## 4. Turn the authentic message into a constant message.

Building a purpose-driven organization never gets done! You need to keep clarifying the organization's purpose for as long as you are there. The one thing that makes it relentlessly difficult is that it involves getting institutions to shift direction—and existing cultures tend to impede movement. As extensions of the culture, managers, too, end up resisting the change. Other impediments are organizational complexity and competing demands. You have to make the purpose the focus of every conversation, every decision, and every problem your team faces. Always ask, "Will this make us better?" "Will this help us to . . .?" When you hold it constant like that, when you never waver, an amazing thing happens. The purpose sinks into the collective conscience. The culture changes and the organization begins to perform at a higher level. Processes become simpler and easier to execute and sustain. People start looking for permanent solutions rather than stop-gap measures that create more inefficiencies through process variations.

When managers and employees used their stated purpose as a filter, it enables them to say no to anything that does not reflect it. When a leader communicates the purpose with authenticity and constancy, employees recognize his or her commitment, begin to believe in the purpose themselves, and reorient. The change is signaled from the top, and then it unfolds from the bottom.

## 5. Stimulate individual learning

As leaders embrace a higher purpose, they recognize that learning and development are powerful incentives. Employees actually want to think, learn, and grow and are not pure economic beings. When a leader gives someone a difficult challenge, it shows faith in that person's potential. The job becomes an incubator for learning and development, and along the way, the employee gains confidence and becomes more committed to the organization and the higher purpose that drives it. By helping employees understand the relationship between the higher purpose and the learning process, leaders can strengthen it. People should be required to reflect on that relationship often. One way is to get them to produce a written document every two weeks describing their purpose, their strengths, and their development. The exercise is not repetitive because the experiences change as do the lessons learned. As employees become more adaptive and proactive, there will be less need for managerial control because they know the purpose and see how it has changed them for the better. You can liken this clear sense of direction to "commander's intent" in the military. If soldiers know and internalize a commander's strategic purpose, they can carry out the mission even when the commander isn't there. This means, of course, that the leader must communicate the organization's higher purpose with utter clarity.

## 6. Turn midlevel managers into purpose-driven leaders

To build an inspired, committed workforce, you'll need middle managers who not only know the organization's purpose but also deeply connect with it and lead with moral power. That goes way beyond what most companies ask of their midlevel people. Managers generally approach leadership like accounting. They are careful in their observations, exact in their assessments, and cautious about their decisions because that is the cultural tone set at the top. Senior leaders are not inclined to get emotional about ideals, and neither are the managers. As a result, employees at all levels tended to make only safe, incremental improvements.

Once you identify your purpose, set out to connect every leader and manager to that purpose. Begin by talking openly about your own sense of purpose and meaning. You may have to invest in a new kind of training, in which managers learn how to tell compelling stories that convey their sense of personal identity and professional purpose. In doing so, they will model a vulnerability and authenticity that is critical to leading with moral power.

## 7. Connect the people to the purpose

Once leaders at the top and in the middle have internalized the organization's purpose, they must help frontline employees see how it connects with their day-to-day tasks. But a top-down mandate does not work. Employees need to help drive this process because then the purpose is more likely to permeate the culture, shaping behavior even when managers aren't right there to watch how people are handling things. You can start by getting employees to share their own accounts of how they are making a difference. One strategy is to get employees to create posters that would answer the question, "What do I do at . . ." while capturing their passion and connecting it to the organization's purpose. They can create a purpose-driven headline and an accompanying clarifying statement.

KPMG ran this as an internal competition and received more than 42,000 submissions. Their purpose is "Inspire Confidence.

Empower Change." Among the submissions were the headline, "I combat terrorism" and clarifying statement, "KPMG helps scores of financial institutions prevent money laundering, keeping financial resources out of the hands of terrorists and criminals."

## 8. Unleash the positive energizers

Every organization has a pool of change agents that usually goes untapped. We refer to this pool as the network of positive energizers. Spread randomly throughout the organization are mature, purpose-driven people with an optimistic orientation. They naturally inspire others. They're open and willing to take initiative. Once enlisted, they can assist with every step of the cultural change. These people are easy to identify, and others trust them. Typically, at an initial meeting, senior leaders invite network members to become involved in the design and execution of the change process. Regular meetings are scheduled. The energizers go out, share ideas, and return with feedback and new ideas. They're willing to tell the truth and openly challenge assumptions.

## Massive Transformative Purpose (MTP)

Eradicating diseases, mastering flight, near-instant global communication, going to the moon—humans have developed a taste for making the impossible possible. Though we still face a daunting list of global challenges, we've learned that science and technology can uncover big solutions. But mind-blowing breakthroughs don't just happen. They take teams of bright and dedicated people chipping away at the problem day and night. They take a huge amount of motivation, toil, and at least a few failures. To solve our biggest problems, we need people to undertake big tasks. But what drives someone to take on such a difficult, uncertain process and stick with it? There's a name for this breed of motivation. Salim Ismail and his co-authors in the book *Exponential Organizations*[23] call this a massive transformative purpose or MTP.

In the simplest sense, an MTP is a "highly aspirational tagline" for an individual or group like a company, organization, community, or social movement. It's a huge and audacious purpose statement, the reason for their existence:

**Massive**: Audaciously big and aspirational

**Transformational**: can cause a significant impact on an industry, community, or planet

**Purpose**: there's a clear "why" behind the work being done. Something that unites and inspires action

My favorite example of an MTP is Aravind Eye Hospital:[24] ***to cure the world of needless blindness***

Setting out to solve big problems brings purpose and meaning to work—it gives us a compelling reason to get out of bed in the morning and face another day. Dr. V and the Aravind Eye Care System are good examples of understanding MTPs. Dr. V didn't find Aravind to have a luxurious retirement or just for the sake of building the largest and most profitable hospital. He was driven by the belief that he could and should eliminate needless blindness in India and across the globe. Making this a reality was his purpose.

---

23  Ismail Salim, "Exponential Organizations: Why new organizations are ten times better, faster, and cheaper than yours (and what to do about it)" (2014).

24  https://aravind.org/.

Aravind's MTP to revolutionize the way eye care is delivered has created a shared aspirational purpose within the organization which continues despite the passing of its founder in 2006.

Notice that Aravind's MTP is:

**Huge and aspirational**: elimination of needless blindness

**Clearly focused**: cataract-related blindness

**Unique to the company**: volume-based operational model (McDonaldization of cataract surgery)

**Aimed at radical transformation**: base of pyramid economic model with more than half of patients not paying

**Forward-looking**: geographic expansion and vertical integration (they manufacture most inputs)

All Aravind employees know the purpose. And not only do they know it, but they are also navigated by it. Because people are highly motivated by the chance to help make a difference. And the MTP is a narrative that awakens a strong inner sense of motivation—unlike external motivators such as money and status—and a desire to help, to do something for others, to help make a difference, and to be a better person. As you can imagine, staff turnover at Aravind is extremely low and the drive to eliminate needless blindness is palpable everywhere.

Other good examples of MTPs include:

Tesla: "Accelerating the world's transition to sustainable energy."

Google: "Organize the world's information."

Red Bull: "Giving you wings."

TED: "Ideas worth spreading."

X Prize Foundation: "Bring about radical breakthroughs for the benefit of humanity."

Clearly, Tesla's goal is not about electric cars. It's much bigger than that, and Tesla is certainly not driven by a vision of becoming the biggest or best electric car manufacturer! At first glance, you'll note that each of these statements is very aspirational, and none state what the organization does, but rather what it aspires to accomplish. The aspirations are neither narrow nor technology specific. Rather they aim to capture the hearts and minds—and imaginations and ambitions—of both those inside and outside the organization. The MTP awakens a strong sense of motivation and a desire to help, to do something for others, make a difference, and be a better person. All Tesla employees know what they go to work to create—to accelerate the world's transition to sustainable energy—and they are reminded of the purpose almost daily, and this is the driving force for both daily operations and innovation.

There is an economic imperative to embracing a massively transformative purpose. The world's biggest problems are the world's biggest markets. An effective MTP can attract customers, and employees and help create a community around a company. It can also shift the focus of teams from a company's internal politics to its external impact. An MTP pushes teams to prioritize big thinking, rapid growth strategies, and organizational agility—and these behaviors all have substantial payoffs in the long term. It also keeps all efforts focused and aligned, which helps organizations grow cohesively. As the organization evolves and scales, the MTP becomes a stabilizer for employees as they transition into new territory.

Although a higher purpose does not guarantee economic benefits, we have seen impressive results in many organizations. And other research—particularly the Gartenberg study,[25] which included 500,000 people across 429 firms and involved 917 firm-year observations from 2006 to 2011—suggests a positive impact on both operating financial performance (return on assets) and forward-looking measures of performance (Tobin's Q and stock returns) when the purpose is communicated with clarity.

So the *purpose* is not just a lofty ideal, it has practical implications for your company's financial health and competitiveness. People who find meaning in their work don't hoard their energy and dedication. They give them freely, defying conventional economic assumptions about self-interest. They grow rather than stagnate. They do more—and they do it better. By tapping into that power, you can transform an entire organization.

So in summary, purpose operates on four major planes: a covenant with customers, a reciprocal human contract with employees, mutuality of interest between society and firm, and the desire to contribute to human betterment. In economists' terms, a company is a network of contracts with everyone—owners, managers, and workers—responding rationally to incentives that produce organizational and wider economic benefits. However, in practice, contracts are incomplete, difficult to enforce, and subject to default. It is through a strong corporate culture that stakeholders are encouraged to internalize the behaviors firms want to create

---

25  http://nrs.harvard.edu/urn-3:HUL.InstRepos:30903237.

and sustain. Purpose is the indispensable means to create such a corporate culture of integrity, crucial to business success.

## From Purpose to Strategy

To safeguard your company at the level of purpose, you must make strategy the servant rather than the master.[26] Most companies have articulated their purpose—the reason they exist. But very few have made that purpose a reality for their organizations. Failure to do this often results in companies being brought down quickly by competitors co-opting their purpose. History is littered with examples of this. *The pepper trade, for example, was disrupted not by a better spice but by refrigeration. It hardly mattered anymore if your pepper supply chain was the best designed and most efficiently run, if your customer base was elite, or if the quality of your pepper was second to none. Your purpose, "preserving food," had been co-opted. All the strengths you had worked so hard to build no longer mattered.* More recently, in the early 2000s, Nokia *was the dominant mobile phone maker with a clearly stated purpose, "Connecting people," and an aggressive strategy for sustaining market dominance. Seeking to extend its technological edge (particularly in miniaturization), it acquired more than 100 startup companies while pursuing a vast portfolio of research and product development projects. In 2006 alone, Nokia introduced thirty-nine new mobile-device models. Few imagined that this juggernaut, brandishing vast resources with such steely determination, could be quickly brought down. In retrospect, it seemed inevitable. Nokia was so immersed in executing its strategy that it lost sight of its purpose. When Steve Jobs introduced the first iPhone as "a leapfrog product that is way smarter than any mobile*

---

26  https://hbr.org/2017/11/the-best-companies-know-how-to-balance-strategy-and-purpose.

*device has ever been, and super easy to use," Apple started "connecting people" at astounding new levels. Nokia's purpose had been co-opted, making its myriad strengths irrelevant.*

Strategies are time-bound and target specific results. Your purpose, in contrast, is what makes you durably relevant to the world. Strategy is an important means to operationalize your purpose. The intrinsic human connection to your purpose is even more important. A company fully operationalizing its purpose would be quintessentially attuned to its world, moving continually toward opportunity, systematically challenging the obvious, and wordlessly yet synchronously making the minute adjustments each situation demands. We can cite no pure examples of such companies, as few seem to grasp the fundamental importance of truly operationalizing their purpose. Elon Musk is one of them.[27], [28] His is driven by "the acceleration of sustainable energy which is absolutely fundamental because this is the next potential risk for humanity." His strategic plan included the following:

1. Create an affordable, high-volume car—electric car (Tesla)
2. Integrate energy generation (solar roofs by SolarCity) and storage (intelligent batteries: Powerwall)
3. Expand to cover the major forms of terrestrial transport (heavy-duty trucks and high passenger-density urban transport in development)
4. Reduce traffic congestion and pollution—autonomous vehicles and vehicle sharing and use of a network of tunnels (the Boring Company)

---

27  https://www.tesla.com/blog/secret-tesla-motors-master-plan-just-between-you-and-me.

28  https://www.tesla.com/blog/master-plan-part-deux.

5.  The final frontier—if all else fails, affordable space travel
    (SpaceX)

Musk's corporate-level strategic approach to reconfigure our
cities, our energy systems, and our impact on the environment is
undoubtedly aimed at his ultimate purpose of ensuring human
sustainability.

Today's economic environment is different. Overcapacity and
intense competition are the norms in most global businesses.
The lines separating businesses have blurred as technologies and
markets converge, creating new growth opportunities where
traditional businesses intersect. And, most notably, the scarcest
corporate resources are less often the financial funds that top
management controls than the knowledge and expertise of the
people on the front lines. Leaders need a fundamental change in
doctrine.

Managers and other business leaders face a dilemma: with
increasingly diverse environments to manage and rising stakes to
get it right, how do they identify the most effective approach to
business strategy and marshal the right thinking and behaviors to
conceive and execute it, supported by the appropriate frameworks
and tools?

When twenty-eighth high-growth companies (average compound
annual growth rate of 30 percent or more in the previous five years)
across three continents were analyzed, it was found that many of
them had moved purpose from the periphery of their strategy to its
core—where, with committed leadership and financial investment,
they had used it to generate sustained profitable growth, stay
relevant in a rapidly changing world, and deepen ties with their
stakeholders.

What's the key difference between low-growth and high-growth companies? The former spends most of their time fighting for market share on one playing field, which naturally restricts their growth potential. And because most aggressive battles take place in industries that are slowing down, gains in market share come at a high cost, often eroding profits and competitive advantage as offerings become commoditized.

High-growth companies, by contrast, don't feel limited to their current playing field. Instead, they think about whole ecosystems, where connected interests and relationships among multiple stakeholders create more opportunities. But these firms don't approach ecosystems haphazardly. They let purpose be their guide. Purpose played two important strategic roles: It helped companies redefine the playing field, and it allowed them to reshape the value proposition. And that, in turn, enabled them to overcome the challenges of slowing growth and declining profitability.[29]

Consider the strategies adopted by Arvind Eyes Hospital whose purpose is to "eliminate needless blindness," which they used to propel their expansion in the broader field of eye health. From an eleven bedded hospital to being the world's largest eye care system, today, Aravind is a network of hospitals, clinics, community outreach efforts, and factories (they manufacture all their inputs and are currently a world leader in the manufacturer of ophthalmological equipment, drugs, and consumables), and research and training institutes in south India that have treated more than thirty-two million patients and have performed four million surgeries. In moving deeper into this larger ecosystem, Aravind did more than just capitalize on a burgeoning industry. It also shifted its orientation beyond services to products, a radical

29   https://hbr.org/2019/09/put-purpose-at-the-core-of-your-strategy.

change for a hospital that had relied on the provision of services. To succeed, Aravind had to build completely different core competencies and devise a new organizational structure. Many hospitals in this dangerously open-ended situation might have failed, but Aravind did not. It was able to pull off a transformation because it ensured that every move it made was aligned with the same core purpose. And it's not done yet: Aravind is now bringing that sense of purpose to efforts to leverage artificial intelligence to improve diagnostic capability at scale, in partnership with Google.

When confronted with eroding margins in a rapidly commodifying world, companies often enhance their value propositions by innovating products, services, or business models. That can bring some quick wins, but it's a transactional approach geared toward prevailing in the current arena. Because a purpose-driven approach facilitates growth in new ecosystems, it allows companies to broaden their mission, create a holistic value proposition, and deliver lifetime benefits to customers.

Strategy today has to align itself to this purpose as well as the fluid nature of the external environment. It must be flexible enough to change constantly and to adapt to outside and internal conditions even as the aspiration to deliver favorable outcomes for stakeholders remains constant. Leaders should think about corporate strategy as a "portfolio of initiatives" aimed at achieving favorable outcomes for society as well as the entire enterprise. Usually, these initiatives will be organized around themes focused on achieving purpose-driven aspirations such as eliminating needless blindness in the case of Arvind or human sustainability in the case of Tesla. Portfolio effects increase the likelihood that some of these aspirations will be achieved even if many others fail.

Mckinsey's three horizons framework—featured in *The Alchemy of Growth*[30]—provides a structure for companies to assess potential opportunities for growth without neglecting performance in the present. Horizon one represents those core businesses most readily identified with the company name and those that provide the greatest profits and cash flow. Here the focus is on improving performance to maximize the remaining value. Horizon two encompasses emerging opportunities, including rising entrepreneurial ventures likely to generate substantial profits in the future but that could require considerable investment. Horizon three contains ideas for profitable growth down the road—for instance, small ventures such as research projects, pilot programs, or minority stakes in new businesses.

## The Three Horizons Framework

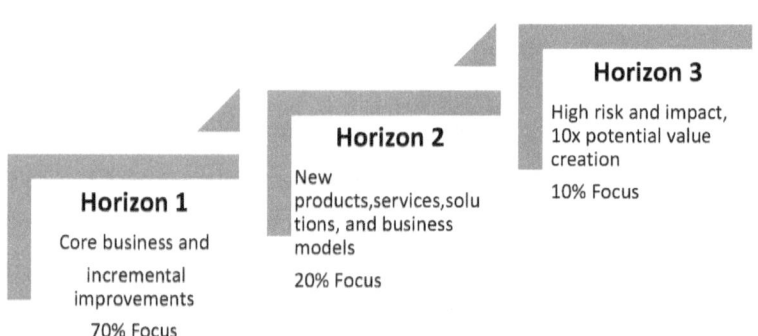

**Horizon 3**
High risk and impact, 10x potential value creation
10% Focus

**Horizon 2**
New products,services,solutions, and business models
20% Focus

**Horizon 1**
Core business and incremental improvements
70% Focus

The first thing every organization needs to understand is that these horizons are worked on simultaneously—you don't complete Horizon 1 and move on to 2 and 3. Part of the objective of this model is continuous growth, and it requires that your team works on initiatives on every horizon. This model gives voice to

---

30  http://growthalchemy.com/introduction/the-alchemy-of-growth/.

the strategic needs of the future while maximizing your current reality. When you put the Three Horizons into practice in your organization, the 70/20/10 Rule is a good way to plan your activities. Seventy percent of your activity needs to be focused on Horizon 1 since your survival today is crucial for getting to tomorrow. Then, allocate 20% of your activities to Horizon 2 which should be enough to account for the failures and missteps your team will experience to bridge to Horizon 3. That leaves 10% of your activities for the research and experimentation of Horizon 3.

## Aravind's Three Horizon Business Strategy Approach

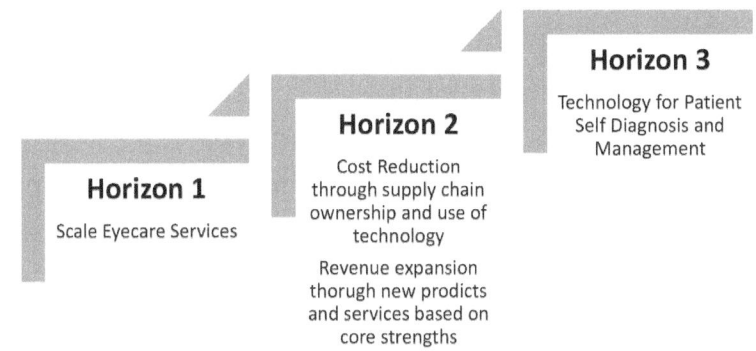

**Horizon 3**
Technology for Patient Self Diagnosis and Management

**Horizon 2**
Cost Reduction through supply chain ownership and use of technology

Revenue expansion thorugh new prodicts and services based on core strengths

**Horizon 1**
Scale Eyecare Services

## From Business Strategy to Innovation Strategy[31]

Random acts of innovation rarely pay off. Despite massive investments of people, time, and money, innovation remains a frustrating pursuit in many organizations, especially hospitals. Innovation initiatives frequently fail, and successful innovators have a hard time sustaining their performance. Why is it so hard to build and maintain the capacity to innovate? The reasons go

31 https://hbr.org/2015/06/you-need-an-innovation-strategy.

much deeper than the commonly cited cause: a failure to execute. The problem with innovation improvement efforts is rooted in the lack of an innovation strategy. For any initiative to deliver true value, the effort must clearly align with a company's business strategy. Yet, successful alignment between innovation strategy and business strategy can elude even the best of companies. In fact, companies rarely align their innovation efforts with their business strategies.

Without an innovation strategy, innovation improvement efforts can easily become a mixed bag of much-touted best practices: crowdsourcing, rapid prototyping, R and D teams, entrepreneurial ventures, and corporate ventures, to name just a few. There is nothing wrong with any of these practices per se. The problem is that an organization's capacity for innovation stems from an innovation system: a coherent set of interdependent processes and structures that dictates how the company searches for novel problems and solutions synthesizes ideas into a business concept and product designs and selects which projects get funded. Individual best practices involve trade-offs. And adopting a specific practice generally requires a host of complementary changes to the rest of the organization's innovation system. A company without an innovation strategy won't be able to make trade-off decisions and choose all the elements of the innovation system.

Mimicking someone else's system is not the answer. There is no one system that fits all companies equally well or works under all circumstances. There is nothing wrong, of course, with learning from others, but it is a mistake to believe that what works for, say, Apple (today's favorite innovator) is going to work for your organization. An explicit innovation strategy helps you design a system to match your purpose and specific strategic and competitive needs.

Finally, without an innovation strategy, different parts of an organization can easily wind up pursuing conflicting priorities— even if there's a clear business strategy. Sales representatives hear daily about the pressing needs of the biggest customers. Marketing may see opportunities to leverage the brand through complementary products or to expand market share through new distribution channels. Business unit heads are focused on their target markets and their particular P and L pressures. R and D scientists and engineers tend to see opportunities in new technologies. Diverse perspectives are critical to successful innovation. But without a strategy to integrate and align those perspectives around common priorities, the power of diversity is blunted, or worse, becomes self-defeating.

Like the creation of any good strategy, the process of developing an innovation strategy should start with a clear understanding and articulation of specific objectives related to helping the company achieve sustainable competitive advantage. This requires going beyond all-too-common generalities such as "We must innovate to grow," "We innovate to create value," or "We need to innovate to stay ahead of competitors." Those are not strategies. They provide no sense of the types of innovation that might matter (and those that won't). Rather, a robust innovation strategy should answer the following three questions:

*1. How will innovation create value for potential customers?*

Unless innovation induces potential customers to pay more, saves them money, or provides some larger societal benefits like improved health or cleaner water, it is not creating value. Of course, innovation can create value in many ways. It might make a product perform better or make it easier or more convenient to use, more reliable, more durable, cheaper, and so on. Choosing what kind of value your innovation will create and then sticking to that is critical because the capabilities required for each are quite different and take time to accumulate. For instance, Apple consistently focuses its innovation efforts on making its products easier to use than competitors' and providing a seamless experience across its expanding family of devices and services. Hence its emphasis on integrated hardware-software development, proprietary operating systems, and design makes total sense.

## 2. How will the company capture a share of the value its innovations generate?

Value-creating innovations attract imitators as quickly as they attract customers. Rarely is intellectual property alone sufficient to block these rivals. Consider how many tablet computers appeared after the success of Apple's iPad. As imitators enter the market, they create price pressures that can reduce the value that the original innovator captures. Moreover, if the suppliers, distributors, and other companies required to deliver an innovation are dominant enough, they may have the sufficient bargaining power to capture most of the value from innovation. Think about how most personal computer manufacturers were largely at the mercy of Intel and Microsoft.

Companies must think through what complementary assets, capabilities, products, or services could prevent customers from defecting to rivals and keep their own position in the ecosystem strong. Apple designs complementarities between its devices and services so that an iPhone owner finds it attractive to use an iPad rather than a rival's tablet. And by controlling the operating system, Apple makes itself an indispensable player in the digital ecosystem.

3. *What types of innovations will allow the company to create and capture value, and what resources should each type receive?*

Certainly, technological innovation is a huge creator of economic value and a driver of competitive advantage. But some important innovations may have little to do with new technology. In the past couple of decades, we have seen a plethora of companies (Netflix, Amazon, LinkedIn, and Uber) master the art of business model innovation. Thus, in thinking about innovation opportunities, hospitals have a choice about how much of their efforts to focus on technological innovation and how much to invest in business model innovation.

| Requires New | **Disruptive** | **Architectural** |
|---|---|---|
| Business Model | • Telemedicine<br>• Ridesharing | • Personalized Medicine<br>• Digital Imaging |
| Leverages Existing<br><br>Business Model | **Routine**<br><br>• Next generation smartphone<br>• Process optimization | **Radical**<br><br>• Medical devices<br>• Biotechnology |
| | Leverages Existing Technological competencies | Requires new Technological Competencies |

Routine innovation builds on a company's existing technological competencies and fits with its existing business model—and hence its customer base. An example is Apple's launching more advanced iPhones which have allowed the company to maintain high margins and have fueled growth for decades. It is the equivalent of the proverbial extra blade on the razor.

Disruptive innovation requires a new business model but not necessarily a technological breakthrough. For that reason, it also challenges or disrupts, the business models of other companies. For example, Google's Android operating system for mobile devices potentially disrupts companies like Apple and Microsoft, not because of any large technical difference but because of its business model: Android is given away free and the operating systems of Apple and Microsoft are not.

Radical innovation is the polar opposite of disruptive innovation. The challenge here is purely technological. The emergence of genetic engineering and biotechnology in the 1970s and 1980s as an approach to drug discovery is an example. Established pharmaceutical companies with decades of experience in chemically synthesized drugs faced a major hurdle in building competencies in molecular biology. But drugs derived from biotechnology were a good fit with the companies' business models, which called for heavy investment in R and D, funded by a few high-margin products.

Architectural innovation combines technological and business model disruptions. An example is a digital photography. For companies, such as Kodak and Polaroid, entering the digital world meant mastering completely new competencies in solid-state electronics, camera design, software, and display technology. It also meant finding a way to earn profits from cameras rather than from "disposables" (film, paper, processing chemicals, and services). As one might imagine, architectural innovations are the most challenging for incumbents to pursue.

A company's innovation strategy should specify how the different types of innovation fit into the business strategy and the resources that should be allocated to each. In much of the writing on innovation today, radical, disruptive, and architectural innovations are viewed as the keys to growth, and routine innovation is denigrated as myopic at best and suicidal at worst. That line of thinking is simplistic.

In fact, the vast majority of profits are created through routine innovation. Since Intel launched its last major disruptive innovation (the i386 chip), in 1985, it has earned more than $200 billion in operating income, most of which has come from next-generation microprocessors. Microsoft is often criticized for milking its existing technologies rather than introducing true disruptions. But this strategy has generated $303 billion in operating income since the introduction of Windows NT in 1993 (and $258 billion since the introduction of the Xbox in 2001). Apple's last major breakthrough (as of this writing), the iPad, was launched in 2010. Since then, Apple has launched a steady stream of upgrades to its core platforms (Mac, iPhone, and iPad), generating an eye-popping $250 billion in operating income.

The point here is not that companies should focus solely on routine innovation. Rather, it is that there is not one preferred type. In fact, as the examples above suggest, different kinds of innovation can become complements, rather than substitutes, over time. Intel, Microsoft, and Apple would not have had the opportunity to garner massive profits from routine innovations had they not laid the foundations with various breakthroughs. Conversely, a company that introduces a disruptive innovation and cannot follow up with a stream of improvements will not hold new entrants at bay for long.

So what proportion of resources should be directed to each type of innovation? Unfortunately, there is no magic formula. As with any strategic question, the answer will be company specific and contingent on factors such as the rate of technological change, the magnitude of the technological opportunity, the intensity of competition, the rate of growth in core markets, the degree to which customer needs are being met, and the company's strengths. Businesses in markets where the core technology is evolving rapidly (like pharmaceuticals, media, and communications) will have to be much more keenly oriented toward radical technological innovation—both its opportunities and its threats. A company whose core business is maturing may have to seek opportunities through business model innovations and radical technological breakthroughs. But a company whose platforms are growing rapidly would certainly want to focus most of its resources on building and extending them.

In thinking strategically about the four types of innovation, then, the question is one of balance and mix. Google is certainly experiencing rapid growth through routine innovations in its advertising business, but it is also exploring opportunities for radical and architectural innovations such as a driverless car. Apple is not resting on its iPhone laurels as it explores wearable devices and payment systems. And while incumbent automobile companies still make the vast majority of their revenue and profits from traditional fuel-powered vehicles, most have introduced alternative-energy vehicles (hybrid and all-electric) and have serious R and D efforts in advanced alternatives like hydrogen-fuel-cell motors.

A good example of how a tight connection between business strategy and innovation strategy can drive long-term innovation leadership is found in Aravind Eyecare System.[32]

| Requires New | Disruptive | Architectural |
|---|---|---|
| **Business Model** | **Horizon 2** | **Horizon 3** |
| | Education/training and Management Consulting (LAICO) | Patient Self Diagnosis by leveraging AI technology (Google partnership) |
| | Primary care Vision Centers | |
| | Tele-ophthalmology | |
| | Eye bank | |
| | Lens and ophthalmic manufacturing (Aurolab) | |
| **Leverages Existing** | **Routine** | **Radical** |
| **Business Model** | **Horizon 1** | **Horizon 2** |
| | Expand hospital capacity | Biotechnology Research for new Ophthalmologic therapeutics |
| | Process optimization to scale cataract surgery | |
| | Community outreach programs | |
| | **Leverages Existing Technological competencies** | **Requires new Technological Competencies** |

---

32  https://aravind.org/our-story/.

It's more than 40 years since Aravind has repeatedly transformed and grown its business through innovations. When viewed through a strategic lens, Aravind's approach to innovation makes perfect sense. The company's business strategy focuses on "selling eye care services" with the purpose of eliminating needless blindness. Executing this strategy requires Aravind to be at the leading edge of high volume, low-cost approaches so that it can solve exceptionally challenging problems for a high volume of the base of pyramid customers. Their initial (Horizon 1) focus was performing their core functions perfectly, effectively, and functionally. They focused on scaling up by routine innovation—optimization of the service, processes, and production methods. This allows Aravind to perform cataract surgery in ten minutes, about a third of the industry standard. And Aravind has managed to keep its infection rates low, an average of about 4 cases per 10,000 patients, compared to an average of 6 per 10,000 in the United Kingdom.

Creating a capacity to innovate starts with strategy. The question then arises, whose job is it to set this strategy? The answer is simple: the most senior leaders of the organization. Innovation cuts across just about every function. Only senior leaders can orchestrate such a complex system. They must take prime responsibility for the processes, structures, talent, and behaviors that shape how an organization searches for innovation opportunities synthesizes ideas into concepts and product designs and selects what to do.

There are four essential tasks in creating and implementing an innovation strategy. The first is to answer the question, "How are we expecting innovation to create value for customers and for our company?" and then explain that to the organization. The second is to create a high-level plan for allocating resources to the different kinds of innovation. Ultimately, where you spend your money, time, and effort is your strategy, regardless of what you say. The third is to manage trade-offs. Because every function will naturally want to serve its own interests, only senior leaders can make the choices that are best for the whole company.

The final challenge facing senior leadership is recognizing that innovation strategies must evolve. Any strategy represents a hypothesis that is tested against the unfolding realities of markets, technologies, regulations, and competitors. Just as product designs must evolve to stay competitive, so too must innovation strategies. Like the process of innovation itself, an innovation strategy involves continual experimentation, learning, and adaptation.

# CHAPTER 2

## Organization

*A pile of rocks ceases to be a rock pile when somebody*
*contemplates it with the idea of a cathedral in mind.*
— **Antoine de Saint-Exupéry**

### 2.1. Innovation Architecture

For healthcare systems, the ability to deliver innovative solutions on a sustainable basis requires an organizational architecture optimized for growth and efficiency. Leadership's role in improving efficiency and creating growth today is all about the "design"— design of the organizational structures that lead to agile, flexible cultures that support internal and external collaboration and rapid cycle time innovation. The challenge involves knowing what kinds of organizational designs will best support your business and innovation strategies, and how to instill these as sustainable capabilities.

The biggest challenge facing healthcare organizations is how to foster and facilitate innovation within the context of a large mature business. Organizations that serve established markets face a daunting challenge: managing and growing the core business while concurrently nurturing and supporting new ideas and opportunities. Organizations designed for large-scale production and delivery are typically poor parents for internal new ventures. Starved resources, inflexible infrastructure, and support structures, and leadership support that ebbs and flows based on the health of the larger organization are symptoms of a broader problem— the fact that established enterprises are inherently designed using metrics, processes, and reward systems suitable for mature businesses, not for fast-moving start-ups.

Ambidextrous organizational architectures are a useful and proven model for driving sustainable innovation within a mature business. They effectively balance the appropriation of value from current business activities and the search for a new value from innovations—balancing exploitation and exploration. This approach creates distinct units that have their own unique processes, structures, and cultures that are specifically intended to support innovation. These units are often comprised of one or more innovation teams, which may or may not reside within the larger parent organization. This is a top-level management responsibility and leaders are obliged to make innovation a core (vs peripheral) activity. In so doing, they have to decide the most appropriate way to do it—mainstream and new stream in separate units or within current operations. Generally, the type of innovation activity dictates the level of autonomy with high-risk innovations (Horizon 3) requiring separate skunk works like units while more mainstream and operational innovations (Horizon 1) are embedded within the breadth of the organization.

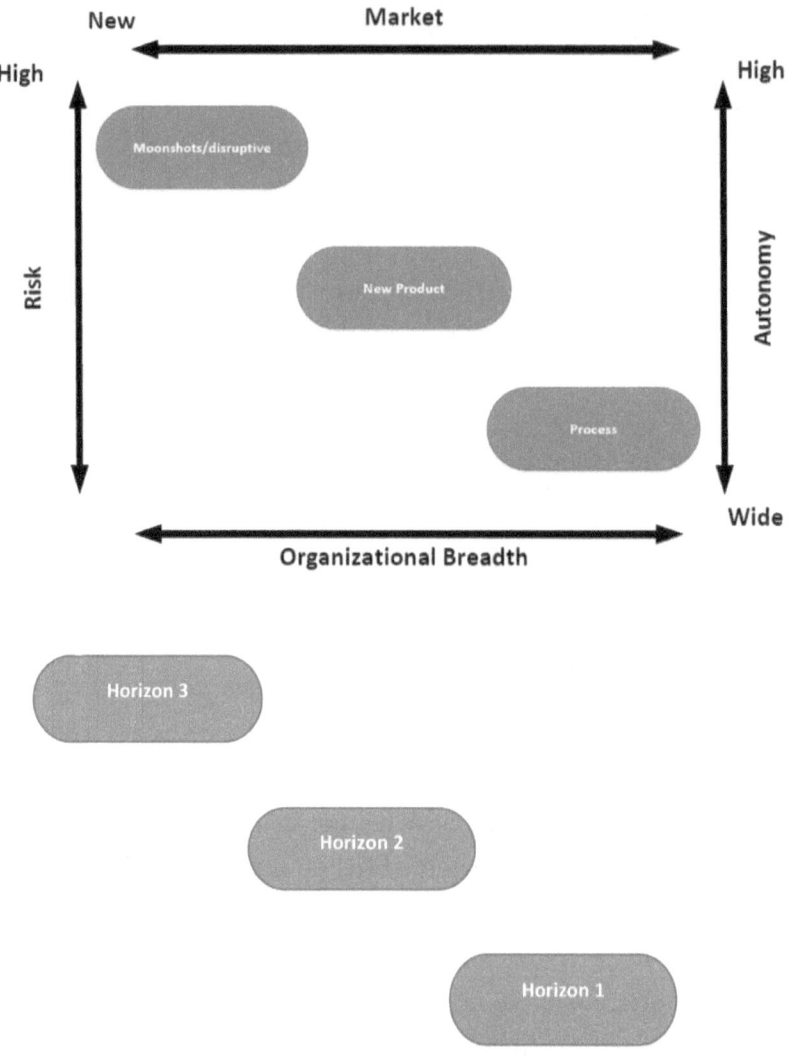

Executive leadership can use the ambidextrous organizational model to create segregated business units for exploring and developing breakthrough innovations (products, services, and processes) while at the same time keeping existing business units intact. Project teams within the new venture are encouraged to form their own processes, structures, and cultures but they are still connected to the rest of the organization through executive sponsors who ensure that no organizational conflicts or competition.

The following figure illustrates two different ambidextrous models. The first is an "innovation incubator" that stands alongside business units. New opportunities are identified, developed, and brought to market by the incubator and either spun out as new business units or folded back into existing units. Alternatively, a business unit itself may create an ambidextrous organization by establishing and protecting a new venture within its own walls.

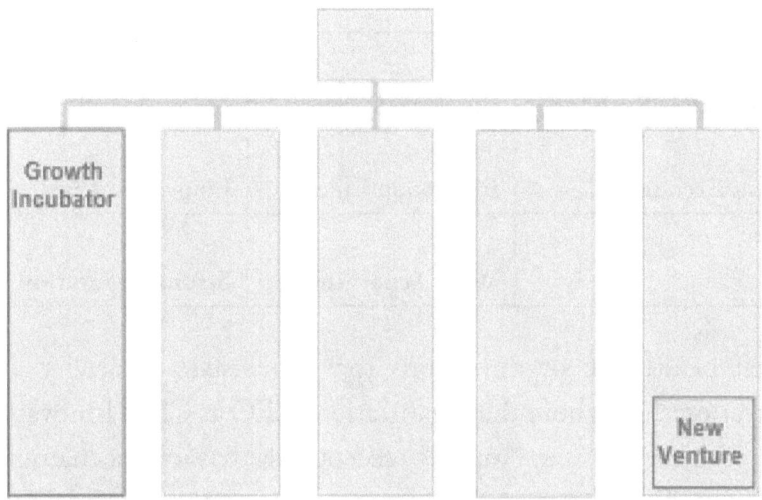

To develop an ambidextrous organization, leadership must possess the ability to attend to already existing products, services, business models, and processes while simultaneously supporting the innovations that will drive the organization's future. Ambidextrous design and management ultimately mean continuing to oversee the core business while concurrently protecting the emerging venture as it evolves and grows. Critical to this leadership function is the ability to afford both the innovation and the operations group equal-opportunity respect because in the chain of creating a breakthrough, the transfer between these two groups is the weakest link. A flawed transfer from innovation to operations is not the only danger. Transfer in the opposite direction is equally important. No product works perfectly the first time. If feedback from operations is ignored by inventors, initial enthusiasm may wane and a promising initiative may fail. Maintaining this dynamic equilibrium between the groups is a critical function of leadership. The key is ensuring the two groups are equally strong and well separated but continuously exchanging ideas and projects in both directions.

| | | |
|---|---|---|
| **Continuous Exchange** | Innovation Chaos | Innovation Ideal |
| **Weak Exchange** | Innovation Failure | Innovation Trap |
| | **Weak Separation** | **Strong Separation** |

When healthcare organizations try to legislate creativity and innovation throughout the organization (CEO as Chief Innovation Officer), chaos ensues. Not every receptionist has to be a champion innovator. Sometimes, you just need them to answer the phone! The commonest innovation trap (bottom right quadrant) however is when leaders create an innovation box in the org chart, rent a separate building, and hang a plaque advertising a new innovation center. When these centers advance ideas only at the pleasure of leaders rather than the balanced exchange of ideas and feedback between the operations team and the "creatives," that is exactly when teams and organizations get trapped, either because no sensible business strategy could justify the innovation (innovation by decree) or because innovations stay parked and never leave because of resistance in the operations team to new ideas. Kodak is a good case in point. They invented digital photography, but the operations team resisted it. The rest, as they say, is history.

Getting the touch and balance right in pursuance of an ambidextrous approach requires a gentle helping hand to overcome internal barriers. If the transfer is forced or under forced, promising ideas and technologies will languish in the labs. The organization will lose the technologies, it will lose the race against time and it will lose the loyalty of its inventors who won't stay around for long.

Another crucial organizational design determinant of innovation success is the management span. Sometimes called span of control, this refers to the average number of direct reports that managers of the company have. The question of what the "best" management span is has been debated in the organizational literature for years. To see how this parameter affects innovation, imagine that you work at a thousand-person company with an average management span of two. That means there are ten levels in the hierarchy (the CEO has two direct reports; those two managers have two reports; those four managers each have two, and so on). When organizations have many layers—that is, a narrow span—promotions are on everyone's mind, "tempting researchers to worry more about titles and status than problem-solving," as the internet pioneer Bob Taylor once noted.[33] Now think of the same company with an average management span of thirty-two. In this case, there's only one management layer between the CEO and the people doing the real work. Promotions occur so rarely that no one thinks about them; instead, they focus on their work. The large group of equal-level colleagues provides "a continuous form of peer review," Taylor said. "Projects that are exciting and challenging obtain

33  https://wiki2.org/en/Robert_Taylor_(computer_scientist).

more than financial or administrative support; they receive help and participation from other researchers. As a result, quality work flourishes, less interesting work tends to wither." Narrow spans aren't inherently worse than wide ones. Narrow is better if you want low error rates and high operational excellence. Wider spans and looser controls are better for experimenting and developing new technologies and innovations.

A Wide Span of Control

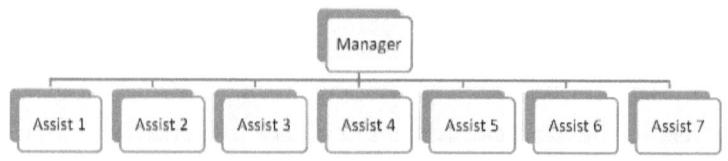

A Narrow Span of Control

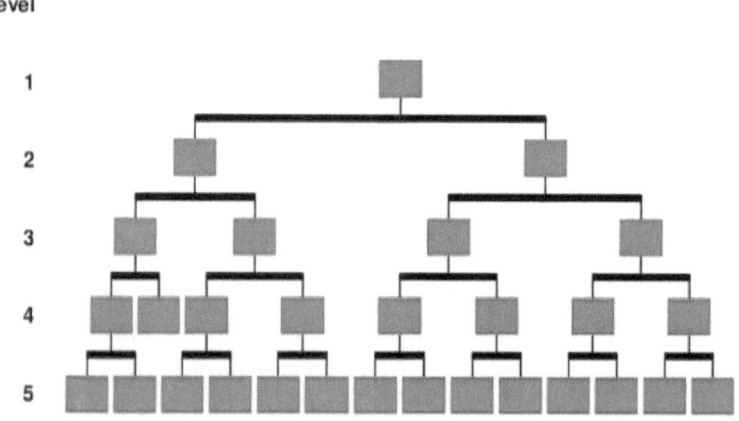

## 2.2 Management Control Systems

It is not easy to make experimentation and risk-taking an integral part of an organization's business practice. Motivating managers and employees to innovate remains a challenge for most businesses. Innovation requires the exploration of new, untested approaches that may very well fail, which flies in the face of the incentives that typically guide business behavior. An organization that wants to encourage innovation must design systems that enable managers to take calculated risks, experiment, and discover what practices and technologies are most impactful and feasible. In addition, employees need to be incentivized to move their projects—not themselves—forward. And although organizational culture has always been espoused as the secret sauce, and to some extent, yes (see chapter 3), it is easier to manage key elements of an organization to foster more-innovative teams even as companies increase in size. Culture still matters, of course, but it's time to pay a little more attention to organization and specifically management systems.

## 2.2.1 Employee Alignment

According to Safi Bachall,[34] there is a certain size at which human groups shift from embracing radical ideas to quashing them. He calls this the magic number $M$. This transition point is not fixed. It is a function of two competing forces, the relative strength of which can be adjusted through variables called control parameters. In organizations, the competing forces can be described as "stake in outcome" versus "perks of rank." When employees feel they have more to gain from the group's collective output, that's where they invest their energy. When they feel their greatest rewards come from moving up the corporate ladder, they stop taking chances on risky new ideas whose failure could harm their careers.

---

34  https://hbr.org/2019/03/the-innovation-equation.

Leaders can tip the balance and raise the value of *M*—ensuring that radical innovation continues in even the largest company—by tweaking four key control parameters. They are equity fraction (E), fitness ratio (F), management span (S), and salary growth (G). Note that none of these are elements of "culture." They are better described as elements of organization design. As the equation below illustrates, a higher M results from increasing E, S, and F (the parameters in the numerator), and decreasing G (the denominator).

$$M = \frac{E \times S^2 \times F}{G}$$

Let's look at how the four parameters work in practice.

## The Four Control Parameters

Imagine that you're a designer at a medical device company, and your job is to develop a better pacemaker. It's 4:00 PM, and you need to decide how you'll spend the final hour of the workday. Should you experiment a little more with your design, or should you use the time to network, currying favor with your boss or other influential managers? In other words, should you focus on project work or on politics?

Such daily choices, faced by pacemaker designers and midlevel workers of all kinds, are what really determine the level of innovation at a company—not cultural changes instituted from the top. The building blocks of innovation are fragile and need broad support; one table-pounding champion cannot take an idea to market. Prototypes must be designed and built, market segments need to be identified, field tests need to be conducted, and so on.

In order for "crazy" ideas to turn into successful products, people across the organization need to be incentivized to invest their time in moving projects—not themselves—forward.

Here's how each control parameter affects behavior:

## Equity fraction

This variable represents the extent to which incentives reflect the outcome of projects as opposed to rank within the organization. Equity fraction ties your pay directly to the quality of your work. If you create a revolutionary pacemaker, the company will probably sell a lot of them, and the value of your equity will grow. Equity comes in two forms, hard and soft. Hard equity includes stock options, grants, commissions, bonuses, and so on. Investment funds pay portfolio managers a percentage of risk-adjusted returns, for example, and professional services firms compensate partners on the basis of the client revenues they bring in. The Chinese appliance maker Haier keeps base salaries low and pays its customer-facing small business units according to their customer sales.

Soft equity—nonfinancial stakes, such as peer recognition—counts, too. If your pacemaker design could be submitted for an industry award, you have a soft equity stake in the success of your project. Whether your equity stake is hard or soft, the higher the fraction, the more likely you are to spend that extra hour on project work rather than on politics.

## Fitness ratio

This parameter involves the relationship between project-skill fit (PSF) and return on politics (ROP): F= PSF/ROP. Economists would call this a ratio between two marginal returns. The numerator is a measure of the rewards from investing time in your project. The denominator is a measure of the rewards from investing in politics.

Suppose you are a highly skilled medical-device designer. An extra hour per day invested in working on your pacemaker might double or triple its value, you might even create a design that will outsell every other one in the industry. The excellent fit between your skills and your project (high PSF) would tip you in favor of spending more time working on it. There would be no need for schmoozing, your triumph would speak for itself. Suppose, on the other hand, that you're not well suited to the projects to which you've been assigned (a low PSF). Your design skills are lousy, and one more hour wouldn't help much. You might as well invest that hour in politics, it might be the best or the only way for you to win a promotion.

In some cases, a poor project fit results from an undermatch: An employee's skills and experience are not up to the task. But an overmatch—skills so far above project needs that the employee is contributing only a fraction of what he or she could offer—is also a problem. Imagine a young Elon Musk assigned to the pacemaker. The project wouldn't offer much of a challenge, and he'd have plenty of time to start politicking. An organization achieves a high project-skill fit when all its employees are stretched neither too much nor too little by their roles.

Return on politics, the denominator in the fitness ratio, is a factor that every employee feels even though it is difficult to measure. It's the extent to which lobbying, networking, and self-promoting affect promotion decisions. This will vary from team to team, but every company will have an average level. Consider two global manufacturers, Company A and Company B. Each has a California office with three vice presidents and thirty product designers. In both firms, a spot opens up for a fourth VP, one of the thirty designers will be selected. Company A is like most firms: The local office will decide who gets promoted. Throughout the decision-making process—which will take nearly a year—those thirty designers will compete to curry favor with the VPs. The return on politics is high. At Company B, however, an independent evaluator who has no ties to anyone in the California office will conduct an assessment and present the findings to an independent group of executives who will make the decision. Since there's little benefit to lobbying, designers at Company B will be likely to focus on their projects and on collaborating well. The return on politics is much lower.

*Management span*

Sometimes called span of control, this refers to the average number of direct reports that executives of the company have. The question of what the "best" management span is has been debated in the organizational literature for years. To see how this parameter affects innovation, imagine that you work at a thousand-person company with an average management span of two. That means there are ten levels in the hierarchy (the CEO has two direct reports, those two managers have two reports, those four managers each have two, and so on). When organizations have many layers—that is, a narrow span—promotions are on everyone's mind, "tempting researchers to worry more about titles and status than problem-solving," as the internet pioneer Bob Taylor once noted. Now think of the same company with an average management span of thirty-two. In this case, there's only one management layer between the CEO and the people doing the real work. Promotions occur so rarely that no one thinks about them; instead, they focus on their work. The large group of equal-level colleagues provides "a continuous form of peer review," Taylor said. "Projects that are exciting and challenging obtain more than financial or administrative support, they receive help and participation from other . . . researchers. As a result, quality work flourishes, less interesting work tends to wither."

Narrow spans aren't inherently worse than wide ones. Narrow is better if you want low error rates and high operational excellence. Wider spans and looser controls are better for experimenting with and developing new and disruptive technologies.

## Salary growth

The average step-up in base salary (and other executive perks) that employees receive as they ascend the hierarchy is another important factor. Again, envision yourself as the pacemaker designer and consider how salary growth might affect your decisions. If every promotion at your company comes with a whopping 200 percent increase in salary, you'd want to make sure that every influential person knows exactly who you are and why you and not your colleague down the hall should be promoted. If, however, promotions yield only a meager 2 percent pay raise, you might as well pour your energy into your project, where some extra effort could earn you a bigger bonus or increase the value of your stake in the company's success. Low salary step-up rates encourage people to use the last hour of the day on work, not on politicking.

Recent academic studies have come to a similar conclusion. One noted that "increased (wage) dispersion is associated with lower productivity, less cooperation, and increased turnover."

Putting it all together, there are many ways companies can adjust the control parameters to increase $M$ and enhance innovation. Here are a few:

## Celebrate results, not rank

To increase the equity fraction and lower the salary growth rate, management must structure rewards to be based more on results than on levels in the hierarchy. Most companies today do the opposite: Not only have base salary step-up rates been rising in the United States, but bonus opportunities at junior levels are tiny or nonexistent (10 percent or less of base salary). Bonus fractions at senior levels, by contrast, can be upward of 50 percent. Celebrating results rather than rank means changing compensation practices—and eliminating (or toning down) widely visible perks of rank such as luxury executive retreats, special cafeterias, favored parking spots, and so on.

## Use soft equity

Many studies have shown that different people are motivated by different things. To some, tangible financial rewards are most important. Others are driven by peer recognition or the desire to help others, or by intrinsic motivators such as a sense of accomplishment and personal growth. Companies should identify and use all the means at their disposal—nonfinancial in addition to financial—to increase employees' stakes in the success of their projects.

## *Take politics out of the equation*

Employees need to see that lobbying for pay and promotions will not help them. One way to do this is to have those decisions depend less on an employee's manager and more on impartial assessments by neutral parties. When promotions are considered at McKinsey, for example, a partner from a different office and preferably a different functional practice interviews candidates' colleagues and clients and then reports back to a group of partners who make the decision. Google uses a similar process. As former HR chief Laszlo Block explains, new managers "are dumbfounded that they can't unilaterally promote those whom they believe to be their best people." The time and expense involved in creating such a system are significant, but it is a worthwhile investment in organizational fitness.

## *Invest in training.*

Companies usually invest in training employees with the goal of better products or higher sales. Send a device designer to a technical workshop, and you'll probably get better pacemakers. Send a salesperson to a speaking coach, and his pitch delivery might improve. But there's another benefit: A designer who has learned new techniques will want to practice them. Training encourages employees to spend more time on projects, which reduces time spent on lobbying and networking.

## *Perfect employee placement*

Designate a person or a small central team to regularly scan the organization for project-skill fit, ensuring that everyone, from new hires to old-timers, is in the right job at the right time. The person or team making assignments should be separate from any particular function to ensure a broad view of the organization. The head of product development, for example, may not be the best person to judge whether a struggling device designer might actually make a great sales rep.

## Fine-tune the spans

Companies should widen management spans and design looser controls for groups in which radical innovation is the goal. Those structures encourage experimentation, peer-to-peer problem-solving, and engagement in project work. Google's former head of engineering, Bill Coughran, once had 180 direct reports.

## Appoint a chief incentives officer

Organizations need top-level executives who are well-trained in the subtleties of aligning incentives and solely focused on achieving a state-of-the-art compensation system. A good incentives officer can identify wasteful bonuses (such as blanket stock options and bonuses based on companywide, rather than group or individual, performance), and reduce the risks of perverse incentives (for example, when an auto dealer's sales goals for service reps lead to overcharging customers), and tap thoughtfully into the power of nonfinancial rewards (peer recognition, choice of assignments, freedom to work on a passion project, and so on). The goal of achieving the most motivated employees for a given compensation budget is as important and strategic to companies as is the goal of achieving the best sales for a given marketing budget (the province of a chief revenue officer) or the best IT systems for a given technology budget (a chief information officer's terrain).

## 2.2.2 Innovation Measurement Metrics

You may have heard the saying, "You can't manage what you don't measure." While there might be an element of truth in the saying, not everything in life, or business, can be measured accurately. Because of the abstract and somewhat uncertain nature of innovation, finding the right metrics to measure innovation can be tricky—not everything that can be counted counts, and not everything that counts can be counted!

While we acknowledge that finding the right metrics to measure innovation can be difficult, it doesn't have to be overwhelming as there are a number of metrics that are commonly used to measure innovation. Choosing the correct KPIs for measuring innovation is important as your goals, and KPIs direct your efforts and actions toward them and help people to adapt their behavior as well as take action to reach those goals. The other side of the coin is that untracked activities are easily forgotten. If you regularly measure your company's innovative output and communicate these measurements, this helps encourage staff to think about innovation accountability on a daily basis and take responsibility for finding new ways of doing things.

Have a look at electronics and whiteware company Haier.[35] Not only does Haier track and measure its innovation in detail over time, it also offers innovative employees the ultimate recognition: having new products named after them. This kind of recognition,

---

35   https://knowledge.wharton.upenn.edu/article/haiers-zhang-ruimin-success-means-creating-the-future/.

combined with the company's approach to measuring innovation, incentivizes each employee to be accountable for innovation, no matter their role. Measuring innovation is a great way to make creativity and invention a core part of every employee's responsibilities, and to celebrate the creativity that exists within your company. The more you know about your innovative outputs, the more you can recognize those responsible for these outputs, which only serves to encourage further innovation.

The most important function of measuring innovation is simple: to ensure you're doing enough of the right activities to reach your goals. Innovation metrics allow you to see if you're doing enough activities, and more specifically, enough of the right kinds of activities to be able to actually achieve your results. It can also help you to guide your resource allocation process, hold people accountable for their actions and responsibilities and assess the effectiveness of your innovation activities. Tracking and measuring innovation can result in major benefits for companies. However, there are also some risks you'll need to watch out for. If you focus too much on metrics, you risk encouraging your employees to hit good numbers, rather than being truly innovative. This is especially the case if you decide to make innovation KPIs part of employee performance reviews. While it may seem like a good idea to rush off and measure everything under the sun, there's plenty of evidence that using too many different metrics can result in a confused and inconsistent picture of company innovation. So start off nice and easy, get the right people on board, and pick just a handful of innovation KPIs, to begin with. Remember, innovation takes time, and not every creative concept can be measured as easily as the next. You wouldn't want to discourage a potentially world-changing idea just because it didn't seem financially feasible in its early stages.

Innovation metrics are typically divided into two different categories: input metrics and output metrics. In other words, "what goes into your innovation process and what comes out of it." Input metrics measure if you're doing enough of the right activities to reach your goals and whether you allocate your resources properly, whereas output metrics measure whether these activities and resources have had the desired impact on your innovation process.

As the name indicates, input metrics, are used for measuring your investments or "The *I* in ROI." In practice, an investment can be for example money, time, or talent devoted to a specific activity related to innovation management. Measuring inputs is a great way to gain insight into how your resource allocation or innovation portfolio matches your strategy and can be considered to also cover metrics regarding the process itself: e.g., how many ideas are passing through to a certain phase.

Here are some examples of input metrics:

- R and D spending as a percentage of revenue
- The number of employees engaging in innovation training or using innovation software
- The number of innovation projects started
- The number of new ideas in the pipeline
- The amount of time senior leaders spends on innovative projects
- Number of new employees in R and D

We think that in general, input metrics are a great starting point for measuring innovation in the early stage because input metrics are responsive. When measuring inputs, you're able to react to changes sooner.

The other end of the spectrum is output metrics, which is a term that is used to refer to your returns, or "The R in ROI." In other words, output metrics measure the results your innovation investments have yielded. As such, they indicate if your investments are actually turning into something useful.

Here are some examples of output metrics:

- Number of new products launched in $X$ amount of time
- Revenue/profit growth from new products
- ROI of innovation activities
- Actual vs. targeted breakeven time for new products
- Royalty and licensing income from patents/intellectual property

In general, organizations are more likely to rely on outputs than inputs. Although outputs are satisfying to measure, they are typically less actionable as they often don't tell you what went well or what went wrong.

In addition, changes in output metrics show only a certain time after the activities have taken place, which especially in the case of disruptive innovation, can be quite a long time. Therefore, it might not be smart to focus on measuring ROI too early. Instead, in the beginning, it would be smarter to assess the time horizon (i.e., how long it will take to break even). In later stages, it makes more sense to pay closer attention to outputs.

To get a more complete picture, it's best to use a mixture of input and output metrics. For example, rather than simply measuring R and D spending (an input metric), you should measure this spending against the revenue generated by products recently released to the market. This combined approach helps to tell both sides of the story: the investments a company is making in innovation, and the results of these investments over time.

One example of this approach is called R and D conversion metrics:[36] R and D-to-product (RDP) conversion and new-products-to margin (NPM) conversion. Their core components—gross margin, R and D, and sales from new products—are not new, but combining them can reveal fresh insight into the relative innovation performance of business units, within an organization and relative to external peers (exhibit 1). The first metric, RDP, is computed by taking the ratio of R and D spending (as a percentage of sales) to sales from new products. This allows organizations to track the efficacy with which R and D dollars translate into new-product sales. The second metric, NPM, takes the ratio of gross margin percentage to sales from new products, which provides an indication of the contribution that new-product sales make to margin uplift.

Two metrics combine R&D spending, sales from new products, and gross margin to shed light on relative innovation performance.

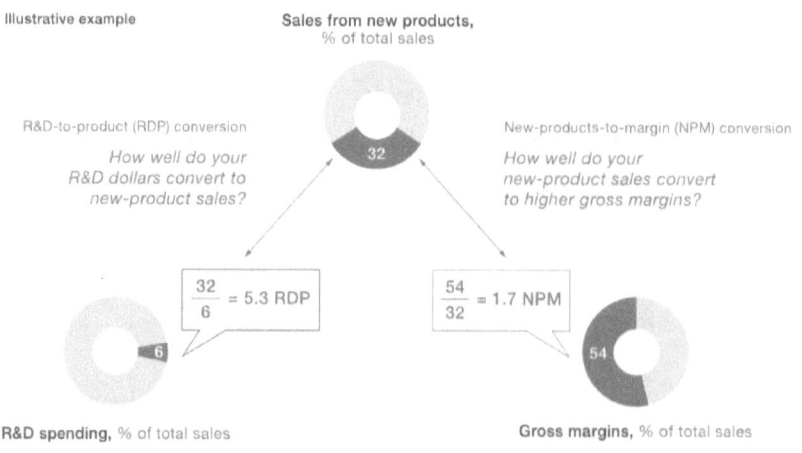

Illustrative example

Sales from new products, % of total sales

32

R&D-to-product (RDP) conversion

*How well do your R&D dollars convert to new-product sales?*

$$\frac{32}{6} = 5.3 \text{ RDP}$$

6

R&D spending, % of total sales

New-products-to-margin (NPM) conversion

*How well do your new-product sales convert to higher gross margins?*

$$\frac{54}{32} = 1.7 \text{ NPM}$$

54

Gross margins, % of total sales

36  https://www.mckinsey.com/business-functions/strategy-and-corporate-finance/ our-insights/taking-the-measure-of-innovation.

Notably, these metrics can be gauged outside in, making them ideal for benchmarking. They also apply on the portfolio level, where the net effect of individual project investments reflects the results as a whole. That broader perspective accords with how senior executives and investors typically consider innovation performance. It's not the most granular way to consider project value creation, and it doesn't aspire to be. In seeking the ideal metric, one should not let the perfect be the enemy of the good. When a business can convert a high rate of R and D dollars to new products, and when its new products flow through to higher gross margins, good things will happen.

As we'd expect, the R and D conversion metrics show that higher spending does not inevitably translate to stronger performance. That should come as no surprise to seasoned executives and analysts. Rather, when we benchmarked companies within select industries, results varied markedly. The R and D conversion metrics also demonstrate—sometimes strikingly—where some organizations are falling short and where opportunities for improvement may be found (exhibit 2). Not every company that scores strongly on RDP is able to follow through to higher margins, and a company scoring above-median performance on NPM may underperform in RDP.

Taken together the conversion metrics can help identify favorable and unfavorable innovation performance outliers.

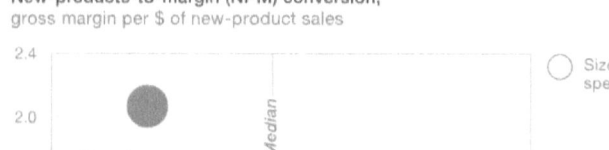

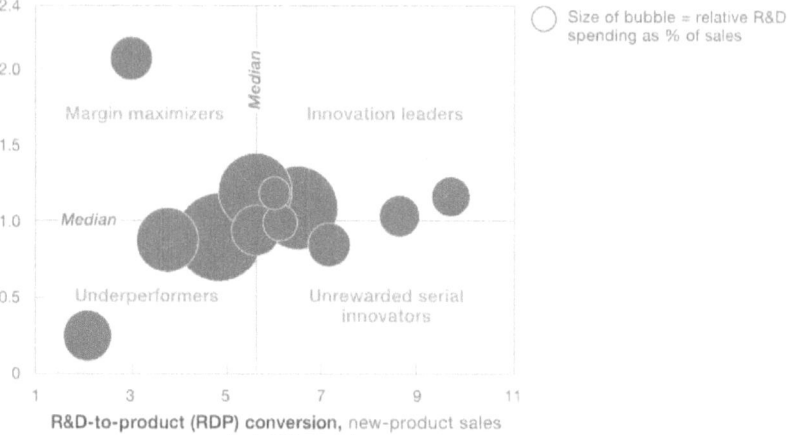

New-products-to-margin (NPM) conversion, gross margin per $ of new-product sales

Size of bubble = relative R&D spending as % of sales

R&D-to-product (RDP) conversion, new-product sales per $ of R&D spend

As we'd expect, the R and D conversion metrics show that higher spending does not inevitably translate to stronger performance. That should come as no surprise to seasoned executives and analysts. Rather, when we benchmarked companies within select industries, results varied markedly. The R and D conversion metrics also demonstrate—sometimes strikingly—where some organizations are falling short and where opportunities for improvement may be found. Not every company that scores strongly on RDP is able to follow through to higher margins, and a company scoring above-median performance on NPM may underperform in RDP.

*Leadership metrics* address the behaviors that senior managers and leaders must exhibit to support a culture of innovation within the organization, including the support of specific growth initiatives. Key leadership input metrics include:

- % of executives' time spent on strategic innovation versus day-to-day operations

- % of managers with training in the concepts and tools of innovation
- % of product/service or strategic innovation projects with assigned executive sponsors

Leadership output metrics include:

- Number of managers that become leaders of new category businesses

*Patient benefit metrics* focus on increasing the outcomes that matter to patients and decrease the costs of delivering those outcomes. In other words, it should be rooted in measuring whether we are delivering value to the patient while minimizing costs. To encourage such a focus, the Centers for Medicare and Medicaid (CMS)[37] is incentivizing the hospitals that provide high-quality, low-cost care with bonuses. Hence, patient experience and quality of care are metrics to consider when determining innovation ROIs from the perspective of the patient. In 2006, the U.S. Agency for Healthcare Research and Quality created the Hospital Consumer Assessment of Healthcare Provider and Systems Survey (HCAHPS),[38] a standardized survey that measures patients' perceptions of hospital care and allows for direct comparison of the patient experience in hospitals across the country. Studies[39] have indicated that there is a high degree of association between patient experience and financial performance, even after controlling for other hospital characteristics that can drive performance. Hospitals

37  https://www.ncbi.nlm.nih.gov/pmc/articles/PMC4910877/.

38  https://www.cms.gov/Medicare/Quality-Initiatives-Patient-Assessment-Instruments/HospitalQualityInits/Downloads/HospitalHCAHPSFactSheet201007.pdf.

39  https://www2.deloitte.com/content/dam/Deloitte/us/Documents/life-sciences-health-care/us-dchs-the-value-of-patient-experience.pdf.

with "excellent" HCAHPS ratings achieved on average 4.7% net margins compared to just 1.8% for hospitals with "low" ratings.

The second metric, quality of care, can be broken down into five key areas: safety, effectiveness, person-centric, equitability, and efficiency.

Safety refers to how safe a treatment is for patients and includes minimizing risk and impact when things go wrong. Effectiveness describes achieving the best possible health outcomes. Person-centric care focuses on the degree to which the needs, rights, values, and preferences of patients are addressed. Equitability ensures fair access to care for all patients. Efficiency describes the delivery and maintenance of the best quality of care.

Creating and driving the effective use of innovation metrics goes beyond simply defining and communicating new measures. Creating innovation metrics requires a strategic and disciplined approach that starts with the enterprise growth strategy and cascades throughout each business unit, division, and group structure. By establishing a "family of metrics" that support the collective innovation imperatives of the healthcare organization, leaders can drive return on investment, organizational capability, and leadership behavior at multiple levels of the organization.

Using metrics to drive and assess growth is not a one-time exercise. As an ongoing tool for innovation management, the approach involves:

Planning: Involving key stakeholders in the identification of metrics to ensure the assumptions about the sources of value are explicit and clear, and metrics align with the firm's strategy.

Monitoring: A way to track metrics against goals to gauge progress and define necessary adjustments to measures and strategies.

Learning: A continuous feedback loop that assesses progress, and engages key stakeholders in identifying implications and new opportunities to support the firm's metrics-driven goals.

The specific process for establishing innovation metrics can include the following steps:

1. Clarify organizational strategic business objectives
2. Define innovation goals to support growth objectives
3. Identify required innovation capabilities for the future
4. Identify desired innovation-related leadership behaviors
5. Identify organizational processes and models required to drive incremental and disruptive innovation
6. Create a family of metrics that support the innovation strategy of the healthcare organization
7. Create cascading metrics that align business units, divisions, groups, and lateral process capabilities
8. Diffuse metrics to drive innovation culture via leadership communication and storytelling, training and development, innovation jams, and social networks
9. Revisit and recalibrate strategies and metrics on an ongoing basis

Whatever the process used, it is critical to engage key stakeholders in defining your metrics that will guide the organization into the future. Learning loops that capture insights gleaned from successes and failures must be integrated into the approach and valued as an ongoing process. And finally, metrics shouldn't be viewed as an end in themselves but rather an indicator of the types of strategic capabilities and behavior required of each and every employee to ensure long-term success and business growth.

## 2.3 Innovation Process

The first sign of a successful innovation program in an organization is the presence of a defined innovation process. The very act of defining and creating a common language around innovation encourages those within an organization to value and critically consider innovation processes. In today's hyper-competitive marketplace, organizations that have robust processes for innovation will lead their industries. Companies such as Google, Apple, and Amazon have been successful at innovating at rates faster than their traditional counterparts because they have found a recipe for successful innovation. Moreover, they have found a recipe for sustainable innovation programs rather than mere spurts of innovation. In too many organizations, innovation occurs by serendipity rather than by deliberate management. Without a process to understand, stimulate, and analyze innovation and an organization's strengths and weaknesses around innovation, most companies rely upon serendipity. Waiting for inspiration to strike is not a sustainable method of securing competitive advantage. Having a well-defined innovation process is important. It makes the voyage from idea generation to product commercialization both efficient and effective.

## 2.3.1 The 3-Phase, 6-Step Innovation Process

There are three key phases (CIE) in the innovation process that every organization typically cycles through: Creativity (Discovery), Innovation (Development), and Entrepreneurship

(Commercialization).[40] Design Thinking links creativity to discovery and business modeling links discovery to entrepreneurship. Business strategy (growth) follows entrepreneurship.

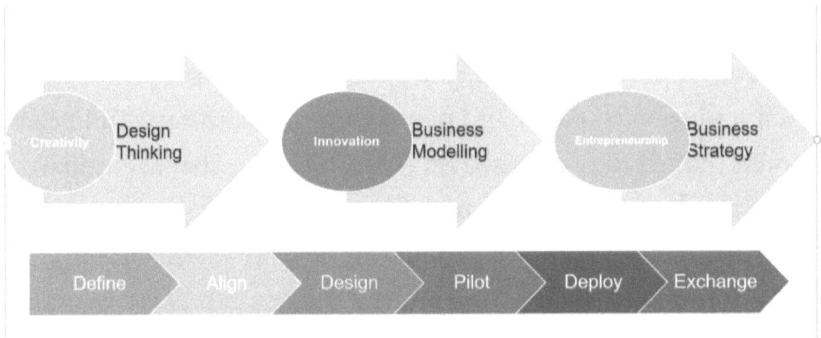

The *Creativity (Discovery) Phase* is the one phase that organizations should spend more time and resources on. It's during this phase that ideas are generated and vetted by potential users, and where teams work to discover whether they're tackling the right problem.

This is where ideation techniques such as brainstorming and prototyping can be used to an organization's advantage. Ideation— the creative process of generating new ideas—is an important part of the design thinking process, in which organizations focus on uncovering the non-obvious pain points their customers are experiencing and developing new products, services, and business models aligned to their needs.

One effective and efficient way to kick off the creativity phase is with an exercise on divergent and convergent thinking. During divergent thinking, there's a free flow of ideas; employees are encouraged to propose and explore as many possible solutions as they can. From there, the team works to "converge" on the concept

---

40  https://www.northeastern.edu/graduate/blog/innovation-process/?msclkid=353
    0f47bc63f11ecbf995a0ee6637025.

they think will most resonate with customers and best achieve the organization's goals. During convergent thinking, teams will often democratize the process by asking each member to vote on the three or four ideas they think have the most potential.

Once concepts are solidified, the goal is to develop a prototype—even if it's just with paper and pen—that the team can put in early adopters' hands to test. Based on their initial feedback, companies might then build a minimum viable product (MVP), or the most stripped-down version of a product or website featuring only the core functionality. By creating an MVP, users can better visualize how the product might work and provide feedback earlier on that the team can use to iterate from. The process enables companies to develop and test concepts in a rapid way for a low cost.

While the terminology might be new, the concept of an MVP is not. Take Henry Ford and the Wright Brothers. They all used iterative prototyping to accelerate the development of their respective innovations. Yet with the propagation of more bureaucratic product development processes, the need to move innovation from idea to development, the discovery phase has become one of planning and analysis, thereby pushing prototyping to the development phase.

We are encouraging organizations to put early prototyping back to where it belongs: in discovery. By the end of the discovery phase, if you did your homework right, you've already tested early prototypes with customers and have a good idea of what your business model is. That's going to better set you up for the development phase.

With the idea solidified and an MVP established, companies can move onto *phase two: Innovation* (Development), where you start to spend real money on design and engineering.

The development phase has changed dramatically over the last ten to fifteen years with the introduction of collaborative and digital design tools and rapid prototyping. Distributed teams, innovation ecosystems, and open innovation efforts enable agile design iteration, faster development cycles, and increased levels of product complexity and performance.

For example, an engineer developing a new medical device can rely on real-time design analysis to make the part stronger and less prone to failure. They can then leverage design tools to optimize the device for additive manufacturing including the 3D printing of final production parts. This can lead to radical designs that couldn't have been achieved with conventional design and manufacturing methods.

Organizations can also partner with firms that crowdsource experts to help solve design problems to gain additional feedback and industry expertise. The benefits of leveraging leading-edge digital design, collaborative tools, and services during the development phase are substantial. This trend will continue as artificial intelligence brings design tools' intelligence to the next level.

During the development phase, depending on your product or service, you also might be

- identifying and selecting new suppliers
- creating the manufacturing and supply chain plans

- establishing a software development kit for third-party vendors
- developing relationships with channel partners

Throughout the process, you should still be gathering consistent customer feedback.

You should be trying to push for as much validation and feedback in each of the stages as possible because it will inspire the next phase. The later you do iteration, the more expensive those changes become. It's more efficient and less costly to make changes early in the process. Over iteration and extending design changes can lead to a detrimental effect we term "back-loading."

At the end of the development phase comes *Entrepreneurship* (Commercialization), where you're bringing your product or service to market. The commercialization process is broken into phases of its own—from the initial introduction of a product or service to its mass production and adoption. As you move through each phase, you'll receive additional customer feedback and will need to regularly refine your offering.

Organizations should explore extended pilot production. Although the launch will be slower, the strategy provides teams with more time to vet any problems and enables them to gain real-time information on market acceptance. Sometimes this can be an extended beta as Google did with Google Glass—good thing that they did it because the result was that the product wasn't introduced in volume. Or as Tesla did with Tesla Model 3. Yes, they had manufacturing constraints but were able to resolve them.

To successfully commercialize your product or service, you'll also need to set a price for the offering and establish a marketing plan.

How will you increase awareness and create customer loyalty? That marketing plan should be adopted across the organization to avoid any communication breakdowns between the marketing and sales departments and the research and development (R and D) or information technology (IT) teams.

Only 39 percent of respondents in a McKinsey survey[41] said their companies were good at commercializing new products or services. When asked what their biggest challenges were, they pointed to the relationship between R and D and marketing, highlighting a misalignment of human and financial resources as well as a lack of processes for manufacturing and introducing innovation.

Establishing an agreed-upon go-to-market market strategy is critical during the commercialization phase. The more streamlined the approach, the more effective the launch, and the more likely it is your product or service will be well-accepted by the market.

These three phases can be further crystalized into six well-defined steps:

1. *Define*—target opportunities that are measurable, visionary, and large impact
   - Opportunity: What problem can we solve?
   - Vision: What will this innovation look like if successful?
   - Patient's voice: Have we sought deep knowledge from patients?
   - Scale: How large of an impact can we have?
   - Metrics: How do we define and measure success?

---

41  https://www.mckinsey.com/business-functions/strategy-and-corporate-finance/our-insights/innovation-and-commercialization-2010-mckinsey-global-survey-results.

- Team: Who is our innovation champion? Who is your operations co-lead?

2. *Align*—make sure the innovation fits within the organization's strategy and engages leadership
   - Fit: Does the idea advance our purpose and strategy?
   - Operations: Is there a credible budget and staffing plan for fill deployment? When do we hand off to operations?
   - Commitment: Is there enough energy around the vision to engage the organization? Will leadership commit to full deployment at scale within a defined time period if the pilot meets the target for success?

3. *Design*—tailor the model to work for the end user
   - Scan: What other innovations have tack this problem with the greatest impact?
   - Partner: Can we find and collaborate with other partners working on similar problems?
   - Expansion: Can we expand our scope to address root causes and improve our impact?
   - Design: Have we convened an innovation team and stakeholders to create the best user-centric design? Have we considered design research, industrial design, and human factors engineering aspects? Can we "rapid prototype" and change quickly?
   - Endgame: What is the business plan and expected returns?

4. *Pilot*—test the innovation on a smaller scale, learn and adjust quickly
   - Learn: Is rapid cycle evaluation built into the plan?
   - Adjust: Have we planned to measure progress and tweak it if necessary?

- Plan for the future: Have we received buy-in from units targeted for subsequent deployment?

5. *Deploy*—deploy the innovation at scale (internally) by handing it off to operations, but continue to watch and learn
   - Transition: Have we handed off to the leadership of operations
   - Track: Do we continue to follow progress? Did we fail early and adjust quickly? Did we have the impact we had planned for?
   - Reward: Have we built in incentives to support and reward innovators?

6. *Exchange*—bring your product/service to the broader market and share what you have learned
   - Commercialization Strategy: Have we explored alternatives? Licensing vs spin-offs vs start-ups
   - Business Modelling: Do we understand the customer segments, channels, pricing, and relationships? Do we understand the cost structure and revenue model? Do we understand supply-side dynamics?
   - Strategic external networks
   - Collaboration skills
   - Partner of choice
   - Exploration of new business models
   - Changing value-chain economics
   - Diversifying profit streams
   - Delivery-model changes and new customer groups

While there's no magic timeline for when you should move through each step, it's recommended you spend more time upfront undergoing the discovery phase. Managing the phases is important and history shows us that front-loading the process is a good thing. The Pillay Health Innovation Feasibility Index below is a useful tool to assist up front to assess the viability of potential opportunities.

| Project | Score 0 - 5 |
|---|---|
| **Stage of Development**<br>Hint: What is the technology's current stage of development?<br>1 = Early stage, researching the opportunity<br>5 = Ready to Launch | |
| **Product Feasibility**<br>Hint: Does the product do what it is supposed to do? Does the technology produce the intended outcome?<br>1 = Unproven concept<br>5 = Proven concept with a workable prototype | |
| **Value Proposition**<br>Hint: How much value does the technology offer customers?<br>1 = Unclear or not obvious value offered to customers<br>5 = Strong, obvious value offered to customers | |
| **Defined Market**<br>Hint: Does the technology have a clearly recognized and defined market?<br>1 = No recognized or new market<br>5 = Well-established, defined market | |
| **Customers**<br>Hint: Are there customers ready to purchase the technology?<br>1 = No existing customers<br>5 = Customers in place | |
| **Competition**<br>Hint: How many competitive technologies are currently available?<br>1 = Many competitors<br>5 = Few or no competitors | |

| | |
|---|---|
| **Revenue Generation**<br>Hint: How long until revenue can initially be generated?<br>1 = More than five years to generate any revenue<br>5 = Less than one year | |
| **Funding Requirement**<br>Hint: How much money will it take to get your idea to the marketplace?<br>1 = More than $1,000,000<br>5 = Less than $50,000 | |
| **IP Protection**<br>Hint: Which IP rights have been obtained?<br>1 = No intellectual property rights<br>5 = Have obtained the patent, copyright, trademark, and/or trade secret protection | |
| **Team Entrepreneurial Experience (ENT)**<br>Hint: How much entrepreneurial experience does the team have?<br>1=Little financial, marketing, and new product development experience<br>5=Considerable financial, marketing, and new product development experience | |
| **Repeat Sales Potential**<br>Hint: How often will customers purchase the technology?<br>1=One time purchase<br>5=Purchase every use | |
| **Market Readiness**<br>Hint: How long until the technology is ready to begin marketing?<br>1 = Two years away from being market ready<br>5 = Opportunity is market ready | |

| | |
|---|---|
| **Reimbursement Potential** <br> (Can we be billed for it?) <br> Hint: What is the likelihood that a third-party payer will reimburse at least some of the cost of using this technology? <br> 1 = No likelihood of reimbursement <br> 5 = 100% likelihood of third-party reimbursement | |
| **FDA Approval** <br> Hint: Will FDA approval be required? <br> 1 = Will require FDA approval <br> 5 = FDA approved or FDA approval not required | |
| **Total Score** | |
| | |
| **Evaluation:** <br> 63–70 = Excellent opportunity <br> 55–62 = Solid opportunity <br> 47–54 = Opportunity needs some work <br> 39–46 = Opportunity has major flaws <br> Below 39 = Very early stage: address major flaws or drop opportunity | |
| | |

# CHAPTER 3

## Competence

*There are two kinds of adventurers: those
who go truly hoping to find adventure and
those who go secretly hoping they won't.*
*—William Least Heat-Moon (Trogdon)*

Competency refers to the knowledge, skills, attitudes, values, and behaviors that people need to successfully perform a particular activity or task. We differentiate competency at the leadership, individual, and organizational levels (culture). It is our contention that a distinct set of knowledge, skills, behaviors, and attitudes are critical for innovative thinking and entrepreneurial action within healthcare. The essence of innovative and entrepreneurial behavior in healthcare is the introduction of a new concept, idea, service, process, or product aimed at improving treatment, diagnosis, education, outreach, prevention, and research with the long-term goals of improving quality, access, safety, outcomes, efficiency, and costs regardless of resources controlled

## 3.1 Leadership Competency

Innovation is a critical tool for leaders in the new health economy and is a fundamental source of value creation in companies and an important enabler of competitive advantage. And yet, despite its importance, innovation is a difficult quality to cultivate both in leaders and in organizations. It is a key survival tactic that companies should use to remain relevant and at the cutting edge of their industry. It is capable of being presented as a discipline, capable of being learned, capable of being practiced.

Leaders with high innovation intelligence (NQ) *maintain a strategic business perspective.* They must be the purveyors of an innovative vision and shape their organizational purpose to reflect that. These leaders demonstrate a keen understanding of industry trends and their implications for the organization. They thoroughly understand the business, the marketplace, and the customer base and are adept at identifying strategic opportunities or threats for the business. An innovative leader does not even need to be the person who creates the idea behind an innovation. Often, she or he simply recognizes a great idea—perhaps devised by a subordinate—and envisions the path that leads to that idea's becoming a reality. Indeed, I would argue that creative genius is less important in an innovative leader than the ability to form a vision around an idea or set of ideas. And once they have formed that vision, they need to be able to share with employees, suppliers, and business partners the vision as well as enthusiasm for turning that vision into a reality. In order to achieve this, the innovative leader needs a powerful imagination, exhibits an underlying curiosity, and possesses excellent communication skills. Developing and communicating a clear entrepreneurial vision is not easy. Such a strategic vision is the mechanism through which those at the top paint the picture of the type of organization they hope to lead—an organization that is opportunity-focused, innovative, and self-renewing. Innovative leaders know that leadership by demand is far less effective at encouraging creativity and innovation than its leadership through motivation and inspiration.

*Link innovation to business strategy*: Too often, innovation is regarded as beyond the scope of strategic management so it happens randomly, haphazardly, and often inexplicably. Innovation should be regarded as an integrated and continuous part of the organization's strategy-making process, rather than as an insurance policy whose appeal varies according to the prospects of the organization's mainstream business. This is a two-directional concept. The two directions are Strategy-Informs-Innovation and Innovation-Informs-Strategy. For the first direction, the key is to make sure you clearly specify the intent of what the firm is trying to make happen in the competitive landscape. This should then guide the use of a systematic innovation process. So for example, if retaining existing 100 percent of loyal customers is a lead strategy, the innovation initiative should focus on current loyalty that recognized and rewarded the fact that customers already understand the technology that made them more efficient and effective at what they already do, and that made them feel very satisfied that they had chosen the right brand, to begin with. For the other direction (Innovation-Informs-Strategy), begin with an innovation initiative to generate a large stock of ideas within a business category. Then map those ideas back into the strategic model to see where they best fit (while remaining agnostic about which strategy to choose). When done correctly, you will see a scatter of ideas around the strategic framework, in a total free-form fashion. Then put your strategy hat on and carefully reflect on the choice of quadrant based on the quality and quantity of ideas within each quadrant. For example, if multi-brand users had the most variety of useful and novel ideas, you will begin to prefer this strategy as a way to make the biggest, disruptive impact on the market. In effect, you let the innovation choose the strategy.

*Cultivate an Innovation Capability*: High NQ leaders invest in the development of an institutionalized capacity for creativity, innovation, and entrepreneurship (CIE). The capability needed is one that allows ideas to emerge from multiple and diverse locations throughout the organization and results in autonomous innovations, not simply planned innovations. Apart from the core responsibilities outlined previously, organizations necessarily have to have a well-defined innovation process in place that spans the continuum from understanding the opportunity and discovering customer needs to generating and screening ideas, prototype development, and testing, running proof of concepts or piloting, scaling within the organization, and commercializing the innovation. High NQ leaders are also responsible for putting in place "pro-innovation" organizational architectures. A pro-innovation architecture is one where the workplace exhibits structural, cultural, resource, and system attributes that encourage innovative behavior both individually and collectively.

*Protect innovations that threaten the current business model*: Organizations tend to ignore, passively discount, actively discredit, or aggressively destroy innovative ideas whose success might undermine the competitiveness or profitability of current operations. High NQ leaders need to selectively protect these disruptive innovations since they will often evolve into engines that drive future sales growth. Such protection frequently involves cocooning or protecting innovative projects during their infancy, a time at which they are most vulnerable to negative intervention from those inside and outside.

*Make opportunities make sense:* How an organization recognizes innovative opportunities is often constrained by how its members think about their business and their respective roles. High NQ leaders should actively seek to expand the radar screen used by the organization to define the companies' opportunities. This might be accomplished by (1) communicating a broad definition of the firm's business (e.g., health vs. healthcare), (2) challenging employees to define the organization's opportunities from the perspective of an innovation model other than that which is dominant for their organization (e.g., market share driven model vs. technology-driven model or process innovation vs care delivery model), and (3) openly and regularly articulating alternative and plausible future scenarios for the organization (e.g., moving toward platform-based care delivery)

*Question the dominant logic:* an organization's dominant logic— how leaders conceptualize the business and make resource allocations—can limit an individual's perceptions and actions to those that conform to conventional and accepted business rules (e.g., inpatient treatment of sick patients). They capture a competitive advantage in the present but may be oblivious to future possibilities. By challenging conventional strategic practices, norms, and mindsets, high NQ leaders frequently identify new products, business models, and strategies. One means of changing the dynamic dominant logic is to make innovation the basis upon which the organization is conceptualized and resources allocated.

*Revisit the "Deceptively Simple Questions":* the deceptively simple questions are those whose answers define the organization and its operations in a very fundamental sense. They include questions like: "What business are we in?" "What is our reason for existence?" "What do our customers value?" "How should we measure success?" High NQ leaders appreciate that there are no single, correct and enduring answers over the course of an organization's existence. They regularly revisit such questions in an effort to identify opportunities for growth and differentiation. They know that Strategic Opportunity Areas (SOAs) lie at the intersection of "WHAT problem will you solve?" "WHO struggles to solve this problem today?" "How might we uniquely solve this problem?" and "WHY are we uniquely positioned to win?"

*Manage ambidextrously:* Highly innovative leaders are characterized by their ambidexterity. They effectively balance the appropriation of value from current business activities and the search for a new value from innovations: balancing exploitation and exploration. This is a top-level management responsibility, and high NQ leaders are obliged to make innovation a core (vs. peripheral) activity. In so doing, they have to decide the most appropriate way to do it—mainstream and new stream in separate units or within current operations. Generally, the type of innovation activity dictates the level of autonomy and risk. High-risk disruptive innovations require separate skunk works like units while more mainstream and operational innovations are embedded within the breadth of the organization. For this to succeed, high NQ leaders oversee both mainstream operations and new stream initiatives. They create direct, unmediated reporting relationships between themselves and those individuals and groups engaged in exploratory, innovation-producing initiatives. In this way, they are able to more effectively balance the resource commitments needed to achieve current and future competitiveness. Finally, high NQ leaders create ambidextrous organizations by setting explicit goals for innovation, for example, by earmarking say 25 percent of revenue to come from new products, services, and markets introduced over the preceding five years. This helps transform innovation from a peripheral activity to a core activity within organizations.

## 3.2 Cultural Competency

In companies, almost everyone involved in innovation management agrees that it is crucial to establish an innovation culture. But what exactly are we talking about? What is the definition of innovation culture? Jens-Uwe Meyer[42] defines the term, on the basis of two hundred international studies, as the following:

*"The social environment that enables staff members to develop ideas and implement innovations."*

Innovation culture is so important. Companies invest significant amounts of money in product development and the development of service innovations. Innovation labs are established to meet the challenges of digitalization and develop innovative digital business models. Organizations set up innovation networks and conduct Innovation challenges. However, despite these efforts, innovation strategies very often fail. The quantity and quality of ideas in idea management and the continuous improvement process are not sufficient. Companies lose competitiveness because organizational innovation and process improvement are neglected. Innovation projects that are managed through an innovation process are not progressing. What is the reason for this? Because a company's innovation culture may not be sufficiently developed. Creating

---

42  https://cdn2.hubspot.net/hubfs/2795213/Strengthening-Innovation-Capacity-through-Different-Types-of-Innovation-Cultures.pdf.

an innovation culture is crucial to innovation management, the innovation capability of an organization, and the implementation of disruptive innovations.

High NQ leaders must create organizational environments that weave innovation and change into their fabric. There are several different terms we hear when we talk about companies that do this well: agile businesses, "learning" organizations, and innovative cultures are just a few. These environments adhere to some key cultural and structural strategies. They actively ***seek out customer recommendations*** and develop a process to evaluate and prioritize ones that have the highest probability of meeting customer objectives. They seek feedback on priorities and customer satisfaction first and foremost and focus on creating a relationship with customers that could be most accurately described as a partnership.

Internally, they create environments where every team member feels safe and encouraged to contribute. They should also feel that they are expected to contribute their best work at all times. This collaboration contrasts with organizations where "special people" contribute more often than others. This happens when organizations move from step-by-step processing to working cross-functionally. All involved departments should remain informed and work simultaneously as a normal course of business. Collaborative organizations create higher-quality prototypes—and they do it more quickly.

Innovative cultures are also characterized by rigorous experimentation. Teams must study problems and put forward well-developed solutions. By shifting to a focus on the scientific method, teams learn to formulate a hypothesis, test that hypothesis, and learn and refine solutions rapidly. Rigorous and rapid experimentation should replace prolonged analyses but requires a defined process as well as mentors and coaches to ensure people had the support they required while learning the new process.

Nimble decision-making is a companion to rigorous experimentation. Team members must make the best decisions possible as quickly as required. These decisions must be open to re-examination as new information surfaces. The need to be "right" must be set aside in favor of continual learning. What was once called flip-flopping will now be called learning. An example of nimble decision-making is combining data-based decision-making with intuitive decision-making to leverage the power of both. Decisions are made at the appropriate point to support the process of experimentation. When experiments are run, participants learn, and prior decisions will be revisited when appropriate and updated.

High NQ leaders (and employees) must value adaptability, flexibility, and curiosity. All of these skills and aptitudes support an individual's ability to navigate rapid change. Employees must remain flexible and focused in the face of ongoing change. They need the capacity to feel comfortable and supported by their colleagues so that they can adapt to planned and unplanned change with creativity and focus. Evolving your organization to become more innovative and change-friendly requires a structured effort to update your culture and the systems and agreements that support its functions. Promoting these key elements are crucial to creating an innovative healthcare organization.

No culture can be innovative without great people, and the demands on innovators have never been greater. So a critical ingredient is the existence of the "right" people. There is a need for creative, risk-accepting, energetic employees who recognize and pursue opportunities and are tenacious in overcoming resistance to innovative ideas. Thus, a major role of innovation-driven leaders is to ensure that the organization employs people with a penchant for innovation and entrepreneurship. This makes the human resource management (HRM) function central to innovation success and therefore worthy of significant investment and elevating the importance of the HRM function.

Apart from hiring the right people, appropriate HRM practices are also directly related to the innovativeness of organizations. Job-related tasks need to be broadly defined with more decision-making discretion and delegation. The increased use of teams also brings together knowledge that hitherto existed separately, potentially resulting in process improvements when teams are on the shop floor or "new combinations" that lead to novel products when teams are in product or business development departments. Increased knowledge diffusion through job rotation and increased information dissemination facilitated by IT may also be expected to provide a positive contribution to innovation performance. Finally, with regard to rewards, personal incentives (financial and nonfinancial) are necessary to reinforce the risk-taking and persistence required when implementing an innovative or entrepreneurial concept. Individual incentives must be balanced by rewards linked to group performance over longer periods of time, so as to encourage cooperative, interdependent behavior.

## 3.2.1 Innovation Orientation (IO) of High Innovative Organizations

Highly innovative organizations are characterized by having specific performance-enhancing attributes managerial philosophies, decision-making practices, and strategic behavior that are highly correlated with both organizational as well as individual success. We refer to this as their innovation orientation which is a six-dimension construct: autonomy, competitive aggressiveness, creativity and entrepreneurialism, reactiveness, and risk-taking, tolerance for failure.

## Autonomy

Autonomy refers to whether an individual or team of individuals within an organization has the freedom to develop an entrepreneurial idea and then see it through to completion. In an organization that offers high autonomy, people are offered the independence required to bring a new idea to fruition, unfettered by the shackles of corporate bureaucracy. When individuals and teams are unhindered by organizational traditions and norms, they are able to more effectively investigate and champion new ideas.

High IO organizations promote autonomy by empowering a division to make its own decisions, set its own objectives, and manage its own budgets. One example is Skunk Works, an official alias for Lockheed Martin's Advanced Development Programs (ADP), formerly called Lockheed Advanced Development Projects. Skunk Works is responsible for a number of famous aircraft designs, including the U-2, the SR-71 Blackbird, the F-117 Nighthawk, and the F-22 Raptor.

## Competitive Aggressiveness

Competitive aggressiveness is the tendency to intensely and directly challenge competitors rather than trying to avoid them.

Aggressive moves can include price cutting and increasing spending on marketing, quality, and production capacity. An example of competitive aggressiveness can be found in any number of "attack ads" in the political arena. Too much aggressiveness can undermine an organization's success. A small firm that attacks larger rivals, for example, may find itself on the losing end of a price war. Establishing a reputation for competitive aggressiveness can damage a firm's chances of being invited to join collaborative efforts such as joint ventures and alliances. In some industries, such as the biotech industry, collaboration is vital because no single firm has the knowledge and resources needed to develop and deliver new products. High IO organizations thus must be wary of taking competitive actions that destroy opportunities for future collaboration.

## Innovativeness

Innovativeness is the tendency to pursue creativity and experimentation. Some innovations build on existing skills to create incremental improvements while more radical innovations require brand-new skills and may make existing skills obsolete. Either way, innovativeness is aimed at developing new products, services, and processes. High IO organizations that are successful in their innovation efforts tend to enjoy stronger performance than those that do not.

How do firms generate these types of new ideas that meet customers' complex needs? Perennial innovators 3M and Google have found a few possible answers. 3M sends nine thousand of its technical personnel in thirty-four countries into customers' workplaces to experience firsthand the kinds of problems customers encounter each day. Google's two most popular features of its Gmail, thread sorting and unlimited email archiving, were first suggested by an engineer who was fed up with his own email woes. Both firms allow employees to use a portion of their work time on projects of their own choosing with the goal of creating new innovations for the company. This latter example illustrates how multiple dimensions—in this case, autonomy and innovativeness—can reinforce one another.

## Proactiveness

Proactiveness is the tendency to anticipate and act on future needs rather than reacting to events after they unfold. A proactive organization is one that adopts an opportunity-seeking perspective. They act in advance of shifting market demand and are often either the first to enter new markets or "fast followers" that improve on the initial efforts of first movers.

Consider Proactive Communications, an aptly named small firm in Killeen, Texas. From its beginnings in 2001, this firm has provided communications in hostile environments such as Iraq and areas impacted by Hurricane Katrina. Being proactive in this case means being willing to don a military helmet or sleep outdoors—activities often avoided by other telecommunications firms. By embracing opportunities that others fear, Proactive's executives have carved out a lucrative niche in a world that is technologically, environmentally, and politically turbulent.

## Risk-Taking

Risk-taking involves the propensity to take bold actions such as venturing into unknown markets and allocating a large portion of resources into ventures that have uncertain outcomes. Starbucks, for example, made a risky move in 2009 when it introduced a new instant coffee called VIA Ready Brew. Instant coffee has long been viewed by many coffee drinkers as a bland drink, but Starbucks decided that the opportunity to distribute its product in a different "make-at-home" format was worth the risk of associating its brand name with instant coffee.

Although a common belief about entrepreneurs is that they are chronic risk takers, research suggests that entrepreneurs do not perceive their actions as risky, and most take action only after using planning and forecasting to reduce uncertainty. But uncertainty seldom can be fully eliminated.

## Tolerance of Failure

Innovation is vital for the long-run comparative advantage of firms. However, motivating and nurturing innovation remains a challenge for most firms. Innovative activities involve a high probability of failure and the innovation process is unpredictable and idiosyncratic, with many contingencies that are impossible to foresee. Innovative activity, therefore, requires exceptional tolerance for failure but not all failures are created equal. A culture that makes it safe to admit and report on failure can—and in some organizational contexts must—coexist with high standards for performance. A sophisticated understanding of failure's causes and contexts will help to avoid the blame game and institute an effective strategy for learning from failure. Although an infinite number of things can go wrong in organizations, mistakes fall into three broad categories: preventable, complexity-related, and intelligent.

Preventable failures in predictable operations can indeed be considered "bad." They usually involve deviations from the spec in the closely defined processes of high-volume or routine operations in manufacturing and services. With proper training and support, employees can follow those processes consistently. When they don't, deviance, inattention, or lack of ability is usually the reason. But in such cases, the causes can be readily identified and solutions developed. Checklists are one solution.

Unavoidable failures in complex systems are due to the inherent uncertainty of work: a particular combination of needs, people, and problems may have never occurred before. Triaging patients in a hospital emergency room, responding to enemy actions on the battlefield, and running a fast-growing start-up all occur in unpredictable situations. And in complex organizations like aircraft carriers and nuclear power plants, system failure is a perpetual risk.

Although serious failures can be averted by following best practices for safety and risk management, including a thorough analysis of any such events that do occur, small process failures are inevitable. To consider them bad is not just a misunderstanding of how complex systems work; it is counterproductive. Avoiding consequential failures means rapidly identifying and correcting small failures. Most accidents in hospitals result from a series of small failures that went unnoticed and unfortunately lined up in just the wrong way.

Intelligent failures at the frontier can rightly be considered "good" because they provide valuable new knowledge that can help an organization leap ahead of the competition and ensure its future growth. They occur when experimentation is necessary: when answers are not knowable in advance because this exact situation hasn't been encountered before and perhaps never will be again. Discovering new drugs, creating a radically new business, designing an innovative product, and testing customer reactions in a brand-new market are tasks that require intelligent failures. "Trial and error" is a common term for the kind of experimentation needed in these settings, but it is a misnomer because "error" implies that there was a "right" outcome in the first place. At the frontier, the right kind of experimentation produces good failures quickly. Managers who practice it can avoid the unintelligent failure of conducting experiments at a larger scale than necessary.

Tolerating unavoidable process failures in complex systems and intelligent failures at the frontiers of knowledge won't promote mediocrity. Indeed, tolerance is essential for any organization that wishes to extract the knowledge such failures provide. But failure is still inherently emotionally charged, getting an organization to accept it takes leadership.

And the standard and such tolerance can be reflected in the principal's choice of the termination threshold for a project. A failure-tolerant principal would choose a threshold lower than the ex-post optimal level, and this tends to encourage innovation from the agent. A failure-intolerant principal would choose a threshold higher than the ex-post optimal level, which tends to discourage innovation pay-for-performance incentive scheme is ineffective at motivating or nurturing innovation.

Steps can be taken by leaders to develop these characteristics and to become more innovative and entrepreneurial themselves. They should consider whether their attitudes and behaviors are consistent with these six dimensions. Are you making decisions that focus on competitors? Do you come up with new ideas for products or processes that might create value for the organization?

From an organizational point of view, it is important to design organizational systems and policies to reflect these six dimensions. As an example, how an organization's compensation systems encourage or discourage these dimensions should be considered. Is taking sensible risks rewarded through raises and bonuses, regardless of whether the risks pay off, for example, or does the compensation system penalize risk-taking? To understand how the organization develops and reinforces autonomy, for example, top executives can administer employee satisfaction surveys and monitor employee turnover rates. Organizations that effectively develop autonomy should foster a work environment with high levels of employee satisfaction and low levels of turnover. Innovativeness can be gauged by considering how many new products or services the organization has developed in the last year and how many patents the firm has obtained. Similarly, is the employee making proactive as opposed to reactive decisions?

## 3.3 Individual Competency

The essence of innovation is action. From a process perspective, an opportunity is recognized, a solution is formulated and tested, resources are identified and acquired, and the solution is deployed internally as well as made available to the external market, adjustments are made, and the innovator eventually exits. These actions must be accomplished in a context that has been characterized as ambiguous, uncertain, stressful, intense, lonely, volatile, exhilarating, and frustrating, among others. Arguably, the ability to achieve this under such conditions demands that an innovator develop certain skills or capabilities. It is our contention that a distinct set of competencies are critical for entrepreneurial action and that they must be developed in concert with more general business competencies.

Employing a multistage Delphi methodology, Pillay and Morris[43] provide evidence for a core set of nineteen innovation competencies. These include both behavioral and attitudinal competencies and essentially enable innovators to successfully navigate the 3-Phase, 6-Step innovation process. They include

*Creative problem solving/Imaginativeness* is characterized by Schumpeter (1942), who posited that creative destruction plays a key role in the innovation process. Innovators who start something are engaged in a process of creative imagination in which opportunities are exploited by continuously combining resources in new ways.

*Cross-disciplinary knowledge* refers to an understanding of the connections, interrelations, and interactions between different fields of knowledge.

*Understanding of healthcare systems* entails having a firm grasp of the various components of the health system and an understanding of the major issues faced by the stakeholders.

*Opportunity recognition* pertains to one's ability to scan and search for new information, connect the dots between incidents that appear to be unrelated to limited cues, and recognize patterns or ideas that suggest potential opportunities in the myriad cues or signals that they receive.

*Assessing the feasibility of an opportunity* emphasizes the need for innovators to make evaluations or judgments on whether emerging

---

43   https://www.ingentaconnect.com/contentone/aupha/hae/2016/00000033/000 00003/art00004?mimetype=application%2fpdf&msclkid=6065727bca4811eca 010006f785a7451#expand/ collapse.

information or changes would lead to viable opportunities with impact and profit potential.

*Design thinking* is a human-centered, prototype-driven process for innovation that can be applied to a product, service, and business design. It is the process of questioning, observing, and experimenting so that you can become better equipped to capture valuable information and develop new business ideas. It requires experimentation in order to understand how things work, test new business ideas or different approaches, and look for valuable insights that may emerge in the process. It includes design research, industrial design, and human factors engineering.

*Business Modelling* is the conceptual structure supporting the viability of a business, including its value proposition, supply dynamics, demand-side dynamics, cost structure, and revenue model.

*Resource leveraging/Bootstrapping* describes the need to overcome resource constraints by leveraging resources from others. It also reflects a tendency for innovators to demonstrate an inclination toward effectual rather than causal reasoning in bringing together unique resource combinations.

*Risk management/mitigation* involves the systematic monitoring, assessing, hedging, transferring, and/or exploiting multifaceted risks encountered as an innovation initiative unfolds. Risk-aversive attitudes discourage individuals from innovative activities (Cramera, et al., 2002) while successful entrepreneurs are willing to first recognize and bear the uncertainty or risk needed to take entrepreneurial actions, and are able to manage risk rather than simply trying to avoid risk.

*Guerrilla skills* is a label adapted from a warfare context, describing approaches that center on clever ways to take advantage of one's surroundings, do more with less, rely upon unconventional tactics, and utilize resources not recognized by others in accomplishing tasks within entrepreneurial firms.

*Conveying a compelling vision/seeing the future* reflects an individual's proclivity for effective communication where he or she can translate his or her vision into condensed, clear, and intriguing messages to important stakeholders.

*Ability to maintain focus yet adapt* speaks to the entrepreneurial experience. This can include considerable ambiguity and uncertainty, significant obstacles, the ongoing emergence of new opportunities, and continuous change in circumstances (Morris, et al., 2012). The entrepreneur must continuously adapt, change, modify, and switch while maintaining a self-regulated focus in the midst of volatile conditions.

*Change management* is the ability to understand and manage driving forces, visions, and processes that fuel large-scale transformation. Information management is the collection and management of information from one or more sources and the distribution of that information to one or more audiences.

*Behavioral economics* refers to an understanding of psychological, social, cognitive, and emotional factors on the economic decisions of individuals and institutions, and the consequences for market prices, returns, and resource allocation. It is the understanding that drives decision-making.

Creativity and imagination, opportunity recognition, understanding of healthcare systems, cross-disciplinary knowledge, information management, vision-based competencies, and behavioral economics are key tasks associated with environmental scanning. These competencies may be developed by encouraging employees to read trade journals, stay abreast of industry trends, have industry mentors, and conduct interviews with established innovators to understand how they recognized their own opportunities. Similarly, opportunity assessment and risk-mitigation competencies in which employees might be tasked with conducting feasibility analyses and risk assessments. Finally, the development of resource leveraging, design thinking, guerilla skills, building and using networks, teamwork and collaboration, and change-management skills which enable innovators to respond in tangible ways to the opportunities may be enhanced by getting individuals to develop business models or plans by using elevator pitches or constructing mock innovation-related tasks or simulations. All of these competencies provide individuals with the skills to recognize opportunities, conceptualize solutions, and successfully execute them. When it comes to innovation, healthcare presents a number of unique challenges. Does the proposed innovation address a real problem that meets market needs? Is there adequate access to the required resources? Does it meet legal requirements? Does it suit the varied needs and interests of key stakeholder groups? It is therefore no surprise that tenacity, resilience, and self-efficacy are significant attitudinal skills important to successfully innovate in healthcare. These can be developed by creating deliverables that are extremely difficult for individuals to perform. Resultant failures or difficulties provide opportunities to teach students how to respond to these stumbling blocks, how to analyze what caused them, and ultimately about the need to persist and endure in order to achieve lofty goals.

# CHAPTER 4

## Linkages

*Many ideas grow better when transplanted into
another mind than the one where they sprang up.*
*—Oliver Wendell Holmes*

Diverse perspectives are critical to successful innovation. But without
a strategy to integrate and align those perspectives around common
priorities, the power of diversity is blunted, or worse, becomes self-
defeating. For many organizations, structuring, managing, and
measuring innovation can be one of the firm's greatest challenges.
Establishing governing processes for conventional functions is
straightforward when compared to organizing for innovation and
growth. But there is a solution—collaboration. Collaboration
allows organizations to bring their best thinking to bear on a
problem, and it's the wellspring of the invention. But how can
leaders facilitate this? Cross-boundary interfaces between different
parts of an organization are called linkages: mechanisms that
identify how individuals and departments within an organization
work together outside of the established formal structure. In a
smaller, less complex organization, linkages are easier to facilitate,
and it often happens organically. In a big company with huge

departments and multinational offices, people often don't know who has expertise in specific tasks or where to go for information or decisions, so linkages become an integral consideration in organization design. By taking the time to plan the linkages, you can avoid wasting resources and energy trying to constantly adjust your formal structure to deal with what could easily be addressed through your company's informal structure.

## 5.1 Internal linkages

Innovation at scale is best achieved when decision-making is delegated to agile, cross-functional teams "with high levels of autonomy." To encourage wider collaboration, companies must tear down information silos. Open information sharing inside companies can take many forms.

### 5.0.1 Innovation Councils

With so much going on in various business units, executive management often lacks a macro view of the various levels of activity and resource investment. Sometimes, several different groups may be pursuing similar opportunities yet operating in a vacuum. Equally, various ad hoc activities may be underway without a clear connection to corporate strategy. This lack of oversight costs the organization unnecessary expenditures of time, money, and human capital, and creates a lack of synergy that could severely inhibit time-to-market. Well-intentioned, yet disparate activities must be coordinated for the enterprise to maximize value.

An innovation council is a governance structure for coordinating and maximizing cross-enterprise innovation. It is a small, cross-functional governance body of senior managers that enables cross-business/function/geography decision-making and coordination. Innovation councils ensure that innovation-related activities in various parts of the organization are strategically aligned and coordinated, and are supported by appropriate processes and resources. From a leadership standpoint, council members' roles involve removing internal roadblocks so that enterprise innovation can be effectively managed.

Made up of senior manager representatives from various business units and functions, innovation councils are responsible for strategic choices as to where, when, and how the enterprise will pursue growth. They meet on a scheduled basis (e.g., quarterly) with a specific capability-building agenda such as the development of innovation metrics, the development of coordination processes across units, or the development of appropriate culture and reward mechanisms.

The following figure illustrates how individuals from different business units participate in an innovation council.

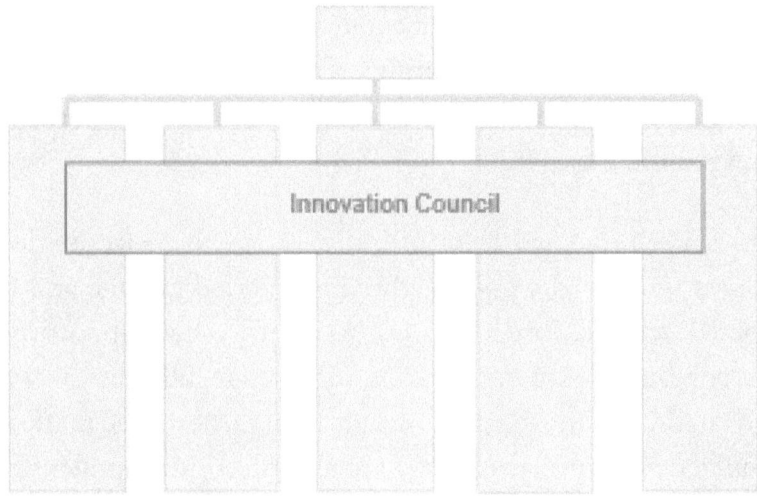

When creating an innovation council, the following must be considered:

- What is the council's charter, responsibilities, deliverables, and metrics?
- How often will the council meet? What is the output of its discussions and decisions?
- Decision rights: what kinds of decisions will the council make/not make?
- What are its operating principles?

## 5.1.2 Cross Group Solutions Teams

How can a large organization with discrete, independently-operating business units successfully identify and pursue opportunities that lie between organizational boundaries? Since business units are focused on their delivering against their own metrics, there is often no accountability or incentive to look for "new growth" opportunities that often fall through the cracks. If an organization suspects that it could be missing a potential growth area, it has the option of creating a Cross Group Solutions Team, an innovative approach for pursuing new growth opportunities "between the silos."

This is a self-directed team of individuals chosen from selected business units who work together for a period of time and have a specific charter, often looking to identify new opportunities that combine the competencies of discrete businesses. These individuals, (technologists, consumer insights experts, marketers, manufacturing specialists, etc.) are assembled to help identify or pursue white space opportunities for which no single business group has formal accountability. In some cases, the individuals relocate to a single location for the duration of the project.

The following figure illustrates the relationship between individuals who ordinarily report to different business units and come together to form a cross-group solutions team.

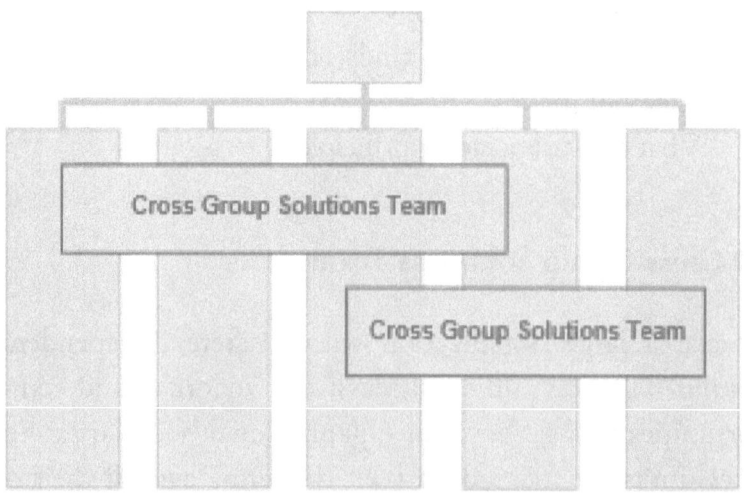

When creating a cross-group solutions team, the following must be considered:

- What is the rationale for investing time in the effort?
- Who will sponsor and fund the effort?
- What are the charter, deliverables, timeframes, and success metrics?
- What skill sets and key stakeholders should be involved in the team?
- What milestones must be met in order to sustain ongoing management commitment?
- Is the organization's current Stage Gate® process appropriate for this kind of approach?
- Will the team be involved in implementation?

## 5.1 External Linkages

Internally-focused organizations sometimes feel they lack the spark of fresh, insightful perspectives that drive their business to greater heights. Companies often struggle to see beyond their own worldview, in which established capabilities, mindsets, and orthodoxies limit their ability to envision and pursue new possibilities. Research and development and marketing groups often find it challenging to deliver truly breakthrough ideas. Fresh thinking is hard to come by if long-time staff always have the same conversations with each other based on common wisdom and orthodoxies. Introducing fresh perspectives, knowledge, and inspiration from the outside allows us to go beyond day-to-day thinking and opens up the mind to entirely new possibilities.

While many companies have historically looked to their own R and D efforts to drive innovation and growth, open innovation proponents argue that today's business logic has changed and that companies today must embrace new strategies for systematically tapping into ideas, resources, and knowledge from the outside. Relationships with external partners such as universities, academic research institutions, government or private labs, and individual entrepreneurs can bring emerging technologies onto the radar screen or spur fresh insights that can be combined with internal competencies to create novel technology combinations that drive new products.

Open Innovation is as much a mindset as a process and challenges an organization's assumptions about the way R and D should be conducted. Below are some of the key differences between traditional approaches and the principles of open:

## Closed Innovation

- The smart people in our fieldwork for us
- To profit from R and D, we must discover it, develop it, and ship it ourselves
- If we discover it ourselves, we will get it to market first
- The company who gets an innovation to market first will win
- We should control our IP so that our competitors don't profit from our ideas

## Open Innovation

- We need to work with smart people inside and outside our company

- External R and D can create significant value; internal R and D is needed to claim some portion of that value
- We don't have to originate the research in order to profit from it
- If you make the best use of internal and external ideas, you will win
- We should profit from others' use of our IP, and we should buy others' IP whenever it advances our own business model

An open innovation philosophy must be driven by an organization's senior executives. In addition to R and D teams, other key internal stakeholders (such as general managers and representatives from marketing, consumer insights, and manufacturing) should be involved to assess feasibility and buy-in from a multidisciplinary perspective. Finally, metrics must be established around open innovation efforts to ensure that the approach delivers the desired

## 5.1.1 Thought Leader Resource Networks

A Thought Leader Resource Network is a model for tapping into external knowledge, inspiration, and strategic relationships. It is an external network of expert practitioners and thinkers that can be tapped at any time. Thought leaders within the network come from companies, universities, consulting firms, research institutions, contract manufacturers, think tanks, and other organizations. Often, under a non-disclosure agreement or as-needed consulting contract, at a moment's notice, they provide specific knowledge, foresight, or recommendations to specific issues, challenges, and opportunities. Because they are all connected to their own knowledge networks, they can also become the doorway to additional strategic resources and relationships.

Formal or informal in nature, this kind of network can be created either by systematically reaching out over time, or coming out of a thought leader innovation panel, which serves as the impetus for establishing the network. Thought leader innovation panel is a one-day client-sponsored event that "stretches" a team's thinking around a particular issue or potential opportunity by introducing the fresh perspectives of external practitioners, visionaries, and provocateurs. By juxtaposing non-adjacent worlds—and exploring emerging trends, it is possible to envision entirely new possibilities and opportunities for growth.

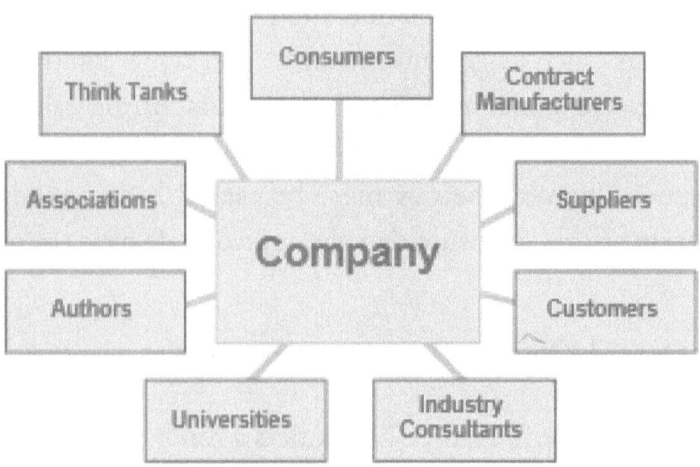

## 5.1.2 Venture Boards for Strategic Innovation

With the movement toward "open innovation," many senior leaders now recognize that in order to drive innovation and growth, entirely new strategies and approaches are required—not just market-driven strategies but organizational strategies. Even with such an appreciation for innovation, however, a big question often remains: how do you formalize an organizational capability for identifying, evaluating, selecting, and commercializing the most promising opportunities for the company?

Organizations such as Procter & Gamble, Johnson & Johnson, Nokia, and Kimberly-Clark have established formal advisory boards focused on bringing external perspectives inside, which ultimately drive innovation and guide strategic investments. Unlike a traditional advisory panel that provides industry and market-related advice, Venture Boards pull together the best thinking from both inside and outside the firm, all within a flexible structure that focuses on a single goal—to discover, evaluate, and drive enterprise growth opportunities.

Venture board membership typically includes the CEO and executive leadership from the company's business units, as well as three to four external thought leaders. The internal members define the selection criteria for choosing the external members, define the portfolio of opportunities to review, and make final go/no-go decisions on strategic investments.

External board members are selected based on their market or technical knowledge, and network of industry relationships that can support potential opportunities. Former CEOs, retired executives, leaders of noncompeting companies, venture capitalists, and consultants can all make ideal members. External members infuse outside perspectives into the board by suggesting additional opportunity areas to explore, providing opinions and advice about the portfolio and proposed investments, and making introductions to outside contacts to advance specific opportunities. The venture board provides a vehicle for the informed exploration of emerging opportunity areas and a format for collectively managing the risk associated with investments in new categories and "white space" opportunities.

The following figure illustrates a common venture board model.

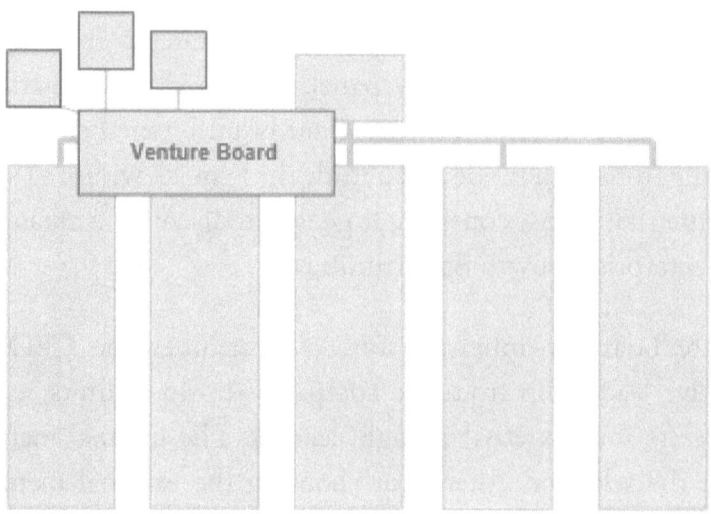

To establish a venture board, executive leadership must define a charter and goals specific to the organization. External members are then recruited and oriented to the company, portfolio, and venture board process. Meetings are usually held quarterly, with defined activities that support specific projects or opportunities occurring between meetings. External board members commit to one-year terms, which allow for rotations of seats based on the evolving focus and needs of the business.

### 5.2.3 Innovation Communities of Practice

Less than 5 percent of employee knowledge is actually captured and made accessible across an enterprise. Given this alarming statistic, how do you best harness critical knowledge to support the strategic innovation of your products, services, and processes within an ever-changing, fast-paced, global environment?

To create value for the organization's internal and external stakeholders, companies must rely on their collective intelligence and shared knowledge to generate best practices. Communities of practice (CoP) are groups of key stakeholders (both inside and outside the organization) who share a passion for an area of knowledge or practice and interact regularly to learn from one another and advance personal and organizational goals. CoPs provide a collaborative framework for this to take place and are a way of leveraging a company's best practices by developing, integrating, and applying knowledge from diverse sources. CoPs ultimately shape organizational culture, foster innovation, and help attract and retain innovation-focused talent.

The following figure illustrates the relationships among individuals across different business units and partner organizations that form a defined community of practice.

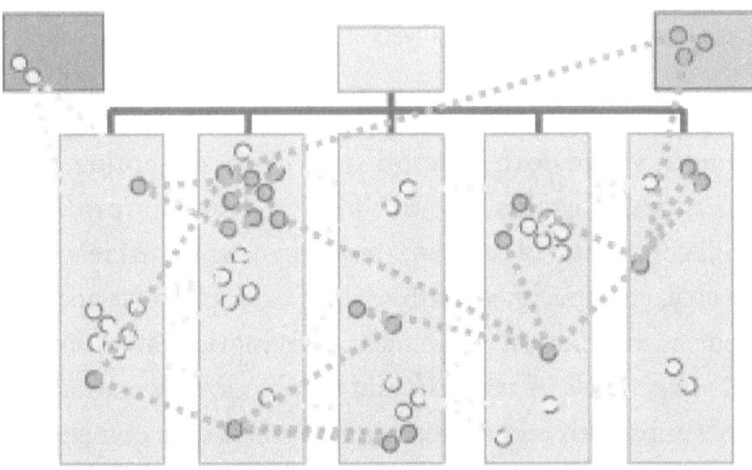

Communities of practice tap into knowledge and resources at the edges of the social networks responsible for driving business strategy, technology innovation, and implementation. They rely on the fact that their cross-functional members belong to multiple communities, which allows for the community itself to stretch its thinking and gain insight into multiple, complementary perspectives. The effectiveness of the community's contribution to innovation greatly depends on the criticality of the community's driving purpose, the quality of top leadership's support, and the collaborative and learning processes and activities that underlie the social interactions that support the community's goals.

As a case in point, the National Institute of Health's business challenge was to drive a large-scale multi-year innovation project that required collaboration between individual functions and across functional groups. Formal meetings and project management tools were too limiting to manage the complex relationships and interactions necessary for knowledge sharing and implementation. A CoP was created to drive collaboration and knowledge sharing to ensure overall project success and resulted in the ongoing identification of critical linkages and dependencies and the sharing of best practices within and between groups.

Disruption will come. The question is who leads it? Health systems need to lean forward and drive disruption through partnerships. Together, we can bring our domain expertise and the full continuum of care into these partnerships to create unique, accessible, convenient, and affordable health products and services for our communities. That means paying less attention to the manic hype cycle of who's in and who's out, but instead driving partnerships with committed big and small tech companies that will accelerate disruption into better, more convenient health care for our communities.

So how do we partner?

There are several key tenets to keep in mind in this area of tech partnership:

*Self-Disrupt Now.* Identify where you must succeed and lead the disruption in the industry either alone or in partnership. This may mean setting up businesses that deliver a better customer experience and business model but may, at some level, compete with existing businesses you own. If you self-disrupt, you have a vote in the outcome. If you don't, you're at the disruptor's mercy. Launch new disruptive businesses and spin out the technologies that you invented to power them so other health systems could make use of them as well.

*Build Internal Capabilities and People.* Recruit leaders from major and up-and-coming tech companies to experiment, build, and scale meaningful technologies. They're also helpful in partnering effectively with both big and small tech. They can translate tech to health care and eventually vice-versa.

*Invest and Partner.* Where the health system is creating value in a relationship, invest in emerging companies to align incentives. Develop a portfolio. These companies will generate a significant financial return upon exit and will deliver far more value via the new revenue streams, cost, and quality improvements. They generate via close, aligned collaboration with our health system.

*Industry Collaborations.* There are many areas where you will not be able to do it alone and need the collaboration of other health systems. Examples include Providence's partnerships with Truveta around data and CivicaRx around generic drugs.

*First Mover Partnership.* If a tech company is doing something disruptive in your industry, first determine if what they are doing will improve patient experience, cost, or quality. If so, try to think of ways to engage, partner, or guide. There is big option value in negotiating early, favorable terms in a disruptive model.

*Embrace Coopetition*: Understand that you will partner in some areas with tech companies and compete in other areas.

# CHAPTER 5

## Conclusion

**Get a good idea, and stay with it. Dog it, and
work at it until it's done, and done right.**
**—Walt Disney**

Strategic and organizational factors are what separate successful
big-company innovators from the rest of the field. It's no secret
that innovation is difficult for well-established companies. By
and large, they are better executors than innovators, and most
succeed less through game-changing creativity than by optimizing
their existing businesses. Yet hard as it is for such organizations
to innovate, large ones as diverse as Alcoa and NASA are actually
doing so. Since innovation is a complex, company-wide endeavor,
it requires a set of crosscutting practices and processes to structure,
organize, and encourage it. Taken together, the essentials described
in this book constitute just such an operating system.

These often overlapping, iterative, and inconsequential practices
resist systematic categorization but can nonetheless be thought of
in two groups. The first is strategic and creative in nature, and help
set and prioritize the terms and conditions under which innovation

is more likely to thrive. The next essentials deal with how to deliver and organize innovation repeatedly over time and with enough value to contribute meaningfully to overall performance. To be sure, there's no proven formula for success particularly when it comes to innovation. While our years of experience provide strong indicators for the existence of a causal relationship between the attributes reported in this book and the innovations of the companies we studied, the statistics described here can only prove a correlation. Yet, we firmly believe that if companies assimilate and apply these essentials—in their own way, in accordance with their particular context, capabilities, organizational culture, and appetite for risk—they will improve the likelihood that they, too, can rekindle the lost spark of innovation. In the digital age, the pace of change has gone into hyper speed, so companies must get these strategic, creative, executional, and organizational factors right to innovate successfully.

Apart from these organizational "essentials," Herzlinger[44] posited that despite the enormous investment in innovation and the magnitude of the opportunity for innovators to both do good and do well, all too many efforts fail. She attributed this to six forces—industry players, funding, public policy, technology, customers, and accountability—which can help or hinder efforts at innovation. Individually or in combination, the forces will affect the different types of innovation in different ways.

The health care sector has many stakeholders, each with an agenda. Often, these *players* have substantial resources and the power to influence public policy and opinion by attacking or helping the innovator. For example, hospitals and doctors sometimes blame

---

44  https://hbr.org/2006/05/why-innovation-in-health-care-is-so-hard?msclkid=7c4
7f32ecfd511ec9ac4c8548837083a.

technology-driven product innovators for the health care system's high costs. Medical specialists wage turf warfare for control of patient services, and insurers battle medical service and technology providers over which treatments and payments are accepted. Inpatient hospitals and outpatient care providers vie for patients while chains and independent organizations spar over market influence. Nonprofit, for-profit, and publicly-funded institutions quarrel over their respective roles and rights. Patient advocates seek influence with policymakers and politicians, who may have a different agenda altogether—namely, seeking fame and public adulation through their decisions or votes.

The competing interests of the different groups aren't always clear or permanent. The AMA and the tort lawyers, bitter foes on the subject of physician malpractice, have lobbied together for legislation to enable people who are wrongly denied medical care to sue managed-care insurance plans. Unless innovators recognize and try to work with the complex interests of the different players, they will see their efforts stymied.

Innovation in health care presents two kinds of financial challenges: *funding* the innovation's development and figuring out who will pay how much for the product or service it yields. One problem is the long investment time needed for new drugs or therapies that require FDA approval. While venture capitalists backing an IT start-up may be able to get their money out in two to three years, investors in a biotech firm have to wait ten years even to find out whether a product will be approved for use. Another problem is that many traditional sources of capital aren't familiar with the health care industry, so it's difficult to find investors, let alone investors who can provide helpful guidance to the innovator.

A frequent source of investor confusion is the health care sector's complex system of payments or reimbursements, which typically come not from the ultimate consumer but from a third party—the government or a private insurer. This arrangement raises an array of issues. Most obviously, insurers must approve a new product or service, and its pricing before they will pay. And their perception of a product's value, which determines the level of reimbursement, may differ from patients. Furthermore, insurers may disagree. Medicare, whose relationships with its enrollees sometimes last decades, may see far more value in innovation with a long-term cost impact, such as an obesity reduction treatment or an expensive diagnostic test than would a commercial insurer, which typically sees an annual 20 percent turnover. An additional complication: Innovations need to appeal to doctors, who are in a position to recommend new products to patients, and doctors' opinions differ. From a financial perspective, a physician who is paid a flat salary by a health maintenance organization may be less interested in, say, performing a procedure to implant a monitoring device than would a doctor who is paid a fee for such services.

*Government regulation* of health care can sometimes aid innovation ("orphan drug" laws provide incentives to companies that develop treatments for rare diseases) and sometimes hinder it (recent legislation in the United States placed a moratorium on the opening of new specialty hospitals that focus on certain surgical procedures). Thus, it is important for innovators to understand the extensive network of regulations that may affect a particular innovation and how and by whom those rules are enacted, modified, and applied. For instance, officials know they will be punished by the public and politicians more for underregulating—approving a harmful drug, say—than for tightening the approval process, even if doing so delays a useful innovation.

As *medical technology* evolves, understanding how and when to adopt or invest in it is critically important. Move too early, and the infrastructure needed to support the innovation may not yet be in place; wait too long, and the time to gain a competitive advantage may have passed.

Keep in mind that competition exists not only within each technology—among drugs aimed at a disease category, for example—but also across different technologies. The polio vaccine eventually eliminated the need for drugs, devices, and services that had been used to treat the disease just as kidney transplants have reduced the need for dialysis. Conversely, the discovery of an effective molecular diagnostic method for a disease such as Alzheimer's would greatly enhance the demand for therapeutic drugs and devices.

A company with a new health care idea should also be aware that regulators, to demonstrate their value to the public, may ripple their muscles occasionally by tightly interpreting ambiguous rules or punishing a hapless innovator.

The empowered and engaged *consumers* of health care—the passive "patient" increasingly seems an anachronistic term—are a force to be reckoned with in all three types of health care innovation. Sick people and their families join disease associations such as the American Cancer Society that lobby for research funds. Interest groups, such as the elderly, advocate increased funding for their health care needs through powerful organizations such as AARP. Those who suffer from various ailments pressure health care providers access to drugs, diagnostics, services, and devices they consider effective.

What's more, consumers spend tremendous sums out of their own pockets on health care services—for example, an estimated $40 billion on complementary medicine such as acupuncture and meditation—that many traditional medical providers believe to be of dubious value. Armed with information gleaned from the Internet, such consumers disregard medical advice they don't agree with, choosing, for example, to shun certain drugs doctors have prescribed. A company that recognizes and leverages consumers' growing sense of empowerment and actual power can greatly enhance the adoption of an innovation.

Increasingly, empowered consumers and cost-pressured payers are demanding *accountability* from healthcare innovators. For instance, they require that technology innovators show cost-effectiveness and long-term safety, in addition to fulfilling the shorter-term efficacy and safety requirements of regulatory agencies. In the United States, the numerous industry organizations that have been created to meet these demands haven't fully succeeded in doing so. For example, a study found that the accreditation of hospitals by the Joint Commission on Accreditation of Healthcare Organizations (JCAHO), an industry-dominated group, had a scant correlation with mortality rates.

One reason for the limited success of these agencies is that they typically focus on process rather than on output, looking, say, not at improvements in patient health but at whether a provider has followed a treatment process. However well-intentioned, these bodies usually aren't neutral auditors focused on the consumer but rather are extensions of the industries they regulate. For instance, JCAHO and the National Committee for Quality Assurance, the agencies primarily responsible for monitoring compliance with standards in the hospital and insurance sectors are overseen mainly by firms in those industries.

But whether the agents of accountability are effective or not, health care innovators must do everything possible to try to address their often opaque demands. Otherwise, innovating companies face the prospect of a forceful backlash from industry monitors or the public.